The CHEATER'S Diet

The CHEATER'S Diet

Daniel Tremblay

Prentice-Hall, Inc.   Englewood Cliffs, New Jersey

Prentice-Hall International, Inc., *London*
Prentice-Hall of Australia, Pty. Ltd., *Sydney*
Prentice-Hall Canada Inc., *Toronto*
Prentice-Hall of India Private Ltd., *New Delhi*
Prentice-Hall of Japan, Inc., *Tokyo*
Prentice-Hall of Southeast Asia Pte. Ltd., *Singapore*
Whitehall Books, Ltd., *Wellington, New Zealand*
Editora Prentice-Hall do Brasil, Ltda., *Rio de Janeiro*

©1984 by

Daniel Tremblay

*All rights reserved. No part of this
book may be reproduced in any form or
by any means, without permission in
writing from the publisher.*

This book is a reference work based on research by the author. The opinions expressed herein are not necessarily those of or endorsed by the publisher. The directions stated in this book are in no way to be considered as a substitute for consultation with a duly licensed doctor.

Library of Congress Cataloging in Publication Data
Tremblay, Daniel
  The cheater's diet.

  Includes index.
  1. Reducing diets. I. Title.
  RM222.2.T7 1984   613.2'5   84-13299

ISBN 0-13-128307-3

ISBN 0-13-128299-9 {PBK}

Printed in the United States of America

To everyone who believes that where there's a will there's a way.

The only way to get rid of a temptation is to yield to it. (Oscar Wilde)

FOREWORD
by
Jacques Cormier, D.C.

What a great pleasure it is for me to introduce this new diet book! *The Cheater's Diet* is not just another diet book; it is a flexible way of life.

Is there any need to emphasize the importance of normal body weight? If you overload a plane it can't get off the ground. If you overload a truck or a car it will not work properly. It's the same with your body. If you give your bone structure too much weight to carry, it will fail you some day. Many times in my practice I have had to advise patients to go on a diet; their back problems were caused or amplified by overweight.

The Cheater's Diet is more than just a listing of good recipes. It gives you important facts about obesity and how to avoid it. It tells you precisely what you should know about dieting. What's more, it reads like a novel. The writing is sincere, precise, and fun to read.

The Cheater's Diet gives you a new approach to dealing with weight problems, an approach that is bearable to every human being. It allows you to return to a normal weight without feeling constant pressure and lets you remain slim while enjoying the good things in life.

If you have a weight problem, if you need dieting, or if you just like cheating, this is your book.

INTRODUCTION

"Another diet book?" I can hear you ask and your second question: "Will it work?"
You bet!
"Is it safe, though?" you ask.
Absolutely.
"Do I know what I'm talking about?"
Yep.

I devised and perfected the Cheater's Diet after close observation of hundreds of men and women who trained at my gym over the years and after my experience as a professional body builder and wristwrestler competing in different weight classes.

There are about 30 million joggers, 20 million body builders, and countless other weight-conscious people in the United States alone. There is a definite need to be filled, and I believe the Cheater's Diet is the *healthiest, easiest,* and *cheapest* approach so far. If you have any medical problems, check with your doctor first to make sure you can follow the Cheater's Diet. If not, you can plan a modified version (with your doctor's guidance) as explained in Chapter 9.

Take a chance on my Cheater's Diet and you will soon discover that living without cheating is only *half* living.

Daniel Tremblay

CONTENTS

Foreword	vii
Introduction	ix
The Dieter's Test	xiii

PART I: WHAT YOU SHOULD KNOW

1.	Why You?	2
2.	The Common Denominator	6
3.	But You've Tried Them All	8
4.	When Three Minus Two Makes Fat	11
5.	How Much Is "Not Much"?	18
6.	Beware of Rip-Offs	23
7.	Shattering a Few Myths	27
8.	In Case You Ask	31

PART II: WHO ARE YOU?

9.	The Dieter's Profile	36
10.	Dr. Pepper's Lonely-Hearts Club	40
11.	The Cookie Monster	44
12.	The Compulsive Eater	46
13.	The Lazy Dieter	49
14.	The Ignorant Dieter	52
15.	The On-and-Off-Dieter	55

PART III: THE SOLUTION

16.	Fasting to Lose Weight............................	58
17.	The French Connection...........................	62
18.	The Cheater's Diet	65
19.	Why Cheating Is a Must..........................	93
20.	How to Cheat Effectively.........................	96
21.	All About Drinks	99
22.	"Smoking" Cellulite Away........................	103
23.	The Modified Cheater's Diet.....................	106
24.	On the Road Again	110
25.	Monitoring Your Progress........................	114

PART IV: FAREWELL FAT CITY

26.	The Healthy Way..................................	120
27.	The Second Most Important Chapter	124
28.	Food for Thought	131
29.	Forty-Six Dieter's Helpers........................	134
30.	Food Supplements.................................	140
31.	Special Instructions...............................	154
	Index	157

THE DIETER'S TEST

Answers on page xiv, but don't peek!

	TRUE	FALSE
1. White eggs have the same nutritional value as brown ones.		
2. One slice of white bread has about the same caloric content as one slice of whole wheat bread.		
3. One obese person out of five cannot lose weight because of hormonal problems.		
4. Calories makes you fat.		
5. Gum has about a hundred calories per piece.		
6. Water contains no calories but does have some carbohydrates.		
7. It's generally harder for a fat person to lose weight than it is for a skinny person to gain weight.		
8. Black coffee contains twenty calories per cup.		
9. Men lose weight more easily than women.		
10. Boiled eggs are preferable to raw eggs.		
11. A soft drink contains fewer carbohydrates than two teaspoons of sugar.		
12. Six ounces of sugar contain twice as many calories as six ounces of animal fat.		
13. As long as you exercise two hours a day you can eat all you want and not gain weight.		
14. Potatoes make you fat faster than any other food.		

	TRUE	FALSE
15. Grapefruit burn fat in your body provided you eat enough of them.		
16. Drinking three to four quarts of water each day will make you lose weight by elimination.		
17. Ascorbic acid is another name for vitamin C.		
18. Canadian lumberjacks are the biggest eaters in the world, averaging 4,800 calories a day.		
19. Amino acids are found mostly in fat.		
20. From a dieter's point of view, eating sugar is worse than eating fat.		

ANSWERS TO THE DIETER'S TEST

Give yourself ten points for each correct answer.

1. TRUE	8. FALSE	15. FALSE
2. TRUE	9. TRUE	16. FALSE
3. FALSE	10. TRUE	17. TRUE
4. FALSE	11. FALSE	18. FALSE
5. FALSE	12. FALSE	19. FALSE
6. FALSE	13. FALSE	20. FALSE
7. FALSE	14. FALSE	

160 to 200: Congratulations! You are well informed—stay tuned. 100 to 150: Good. You know better than the average person but some important facts still elude you. 50 to 90: You are among the average but nothing to write home about. 0 to 40: Where have you been? In the boondocks? Keep on reading, you have a lot of catching up to do.

Some of the above answers don't require explanation; as for the more complex ones, they will be discussed at length in the following pages.

The
CHEATER'S
Diet

Part I

What You Should Know

1

WHY YOU?

We know what we are but know not what we may be. (William Shakespeare)

Who is the fattest human being ever recorded? According to the *Guinness Book of World Records* it's Michael Walker of Clinton, Iowa, who weighed 1,183 pounds in 1971.

Another American, Jon Minnoch, reached the mind-boggling weight of 1,400 pounds in 1978.

And you think you have a problem . . .

Your chances of breaking these world records are almost nil, even if you spend your whole life trying to do so—which is far from your dearest goal I'm sure. However, *The Cheater's Diet* is not a book about medical phenomena; it's a book about normal people who have an excess of body weight—people like you and me. Among obese (extremely fat) people, the occurrence of hormonal or metabolic dysfunction may be one in every hundred. So, mathematically speaking, there's fat chance of your having such a disease (as you will see, it really is a disease).

Many years ago, a friend of mine, Doctor Jean Delagrave, hospitalized a 5'7", 348-pound man afflicted with such a problem. After many tests on his patient, the doctor put the man on a 500-calorie-per-day diet. A week on this treatment and the patient gained two pounds! Within a year, this middle-aged-man died . . .

Americans started a war against fat some 30 years ago. As a result, statistics show we have gained an average of five pounds each, so it looks as if we're losing the battle of the bulge, as a group at least.

Yet some lucky individuals can eat all they want and maintain their normal weight, or at least stay close to it. Why are you the one who stores fat like a bear in summer, no matter what you seem to be doing?

The answer to this simple question is complex. Many factors are involved. Let's try to shed some light on them.

ENVIRONMENTAL INFLUENCES

The first and foremost reason you are fat is the environment you live in.

The country you were born in, the type of job you hold, whether you are married or single, the people you hang around with, these are all exterior factors that have major influences on how fat *you* are.

No matter how you look at it, the one single factor that really makes the difference is the abundance and quantity of food your environment offers you and the quantity you take in. The abundance of food per se is okay, but food processing is something we all have to pay for in the long run. By altering natural food man ends up with concentrated sources of calories (like butter and oils) and with junk food. Junk food cannot qualify as a food because it either has no nutritional value or is too high in chemicals and additives.

Thus if you eat a lot of fat (saturated or unsaturated) and junk food, it's safe to say that your chances of becoming fat—especially after thirty—are very good indeed. Add to this a lack of physical activity and you have the main reasons most people are overweight.

A man who works ten hours a day in a salt mine cannot eat all day long, and he probably doesn't have much energy left to indulge in eating huge amounts of food at the end of the shift. Moreover, he has burned up a significant amount of calories in his labor. Likewise, an office worker who plays racquetball for three hours each evening can't eat during that time, and uses up about 1,500 calories in the process. Yet if that same office worker spent three hours sitting in front of the tube eating on and off, he or she would cram in about 2,000 calories *in excess* of his body requirement; that would be equal to four pounds of extra weight by the end of the week. The problem is people coming back from work and not knowing what to do. They sit in front of the TV set, get brainwashed by publicity and rush to the fridge to satisfy their *psychological* need for food. Let's face it. If you spend six hours in front of the tube each night, there's a ninety percent chance that you are fat. Physically speaking you can separate people into two basic groups: the doers and the lookers. If you're a looker you're probably fat, and if you're a doer you're probably not.

Technology—more specifically, television—has made more fatsos than all the tons of French fries sold in America.

PARENTAL HABITS

From generation to generation, eating habits are transmitted without much questioning, unfortunately. Thus you may say that a basic amount of fat is inherited from your parents. That's another reason why *you* are fat. But you are not alone. About one hundred million people in the United States are overweight. Some of them are fat and others are obese. Some experts say you are obese when you're twenty-five percent above your normal body weight, while others say only fifteen percent suffices to qualify you for the title. I won't give you any figure, but I can quickly spot an obese person in a crowd. As far as I'm concerned, anyone who's extremely fat is an obese person.

I once worked for a friend of my father. The man, who owned a restaurant, was obese. My father was also a restaurant owner but he was built like a prize fighter. One day, my father's friend invited me to have dinner with him and his family, and I accepted. At home, I met his wife. She was also obese and so were his two young boys, who were about five and six years old. That night the menu consisted of pasta, Italian gravy, melted cheese, and garlic bread. After eating the big serving of spaghetti his wife had given me, I was full. To my surprise they all took two or more servings as big as the one I had. Seeing my consternation over the kids eating so much, he explained to me (proudly) that they were used to eating like that since they had learned to walk. After the meal we moved from the table to the television set (where else?). Within half an hour after that big meal, the kids were having chips and soda. That was incredible to me, but it was natural for this family. The parents had inherited this habit from their parents and were now passing it down to their children, who will surely transmit it to their children, and so on and so on.

Unfortunately, fat is a more common legacy today than money.

MEN, WOMEN, AND FAT

The fact that you are born male or female has much to do with why you are fat, or rather, why you are fatter than you'd like to be.

Normally, men have about fifteen percent body fat and women carry around twenty-five percent body fat. For many women in America, the average is closer to thirty-five percent. So we can see that, compared to men, women have an extra ten to twenty percent body fat to start with. Moreover, men have higher metabolic rates and can lose weight more easily; they also have about thirty-five percent more androgenic hormones than women. As a result, men have more muscle and less fat.

If you're a woman, don't let these facts discourage you. Generally speaking, women show more determination in losing weight than men do. Just a look at the new breed of women body builders (who carry about ten percent fat in their bodies) should be enough to convince you that anyone can dramatically improve through a sensible diet and exercise. Finally, whether you are a man or a woman, it all comes down to how much you really want to reach your goal.

2

THE COMMON DENOMINATOR

ALL human beings are born free and equal in dignity and rights. (U.N., Declaration of Human Rights, Art.1.)

If overconsumption of junk foods and high-calorie foods in general is the first direct cause of fatness, why aren't all people who overeat fat? How come the guy next door eats twice as much as you do and stays his normal weight while you're drowning in fat? The answer lies in the fact that *all* obese human beings are born with the same common denominator, namely, a *slow* metabolism. A slow metabolism is the first indirect cause of your fatness.

Let me define that very important word: metabolism. It encompasses the complex physical and chemical processes involved in the maintenance of life. To put it more simply, it's the transformation of living matter within your body. Each group of food is metabolized differently in your system. Sugar, fat, and protein require their own complex metabolic process to be transformed into energy or to help repair body tissues.

Metabolism involves two completely different processes: anabolism and catabolism. Anabolism is the constructive part (build up) of metabolism; catabolism is the degradation of matter (tear down) to produce energy. Those two processes occur simultaneously in your body but with varying degrees of intensity depending on the circumstances.

What does this mean? Simply that in order to lose weight you have to put your body into a catabolic state for a long enough period of time. You do this by eating less calories than you normally need, thus forcing your body to feed on its reserves of fat. A bear goes through the same catabolic state, although at a much slower rate, during its winter hibernation.

Basically, people have either a slow, medium, or fast metabolism. A slow or medium metabolism means that you can gain weight easily and your chance of being fat is excellent. If you have a fast metabolism your chance of being obese is about as good as your chance of doing the Rubik's Cube in less than a minute.

In a way, fat people are lucky. It's easier for a fat person to lose weight than it is for a skinny person to gain it. Many times I've seen the proverbial 97-pound weakling come shyly into my gym and desperately ask if I could help him to gain weight. I would put him on a high-calorie diet, have him eat like a small horse, drink milk shakes by the carloads, and do specific exercises regularly. Despite all those efforts, the man would step on a scale two months later and weigh in at ninety-eight and three-quarters pounds, ninety-nine, or one hundred pounds! Sure, if he stayed on the program for a year he'd probably gain ten or twelve pounds, but as soon as he stopped the forced feeding, he'd invariably see those hard-gained pounds melt away like ice on a tropical beach.

The scenario for overweight people who joined my gym was quite different. Most of them would lose ten pounds in the first two weeks. When I weighed them at the two-month control period, weight loss averaging fifteen to twenty pounds was common.

But who wants to gain weight? you might ask. Well, for one, the man who's six-foot-one and weighs 125 pounds after a heavy dinner is not exactly happy with his body. Neither is the five-foot-six, eighty-nine-pound woman who has to walk twice in front of the sun to see her shadow. Yet if neither the fat nor the skinny person succeeds in that goal of losing or gaining weight, the skinny person ends up the winner because, generally speaking, it's healthier to be thin than it is to be fat. Many diseases are associated with fatness, and obese people often die young. Who has ever seen an obese centenarian?

When you reach the age of thirty, time is not on your side anymore and your metabolism starts to slow down.* This is the chief reason why people are at their heaviest in their mid-fifties or so. Many people reaching their forties are puzzled to see an increase in their weight even though they are not eating more than they did in their early twenties. This weight increase is directly related to age. Right now I'm as old as Jesus was when he died and I know I could easily reach the two-hundred-pound mark if I ate the way the average person does. But I also remember fighting like hell to get over 160 pounds to make the high school football team when I was eighteen. As the years passed my metabolism slowed down, making it easier for me to gain weight.

So, as you grow older, the best thing you can do is to progressively reduce your food intake. This coupled with regular activities is the best way to keep an even, normal body weight throughout your life.

---

*Every ten years or so, your metabolism slows down about three percent.

3

BUT YOU'VE TRIED THEM ALL

There is no failure except in no longer trying. There is no defeat except from within, no really insurmountable barrier save our own inherent weakness of purpose. (Kin Hubbard)

Most diets are doomed to failure. Their downfall is mainly attributable to sheer boredom. Eating tuna fish packed in water until it oozes from every pore of your body or grapefruit until you have nightmares about it can be depressing (like slavery, which is what most diets are anyway). Many diets are unhealthy. They can get you a free ride to the hospital or even a not-so-free one to the cemetery. Not so long ago some people died after extensively using a liquid protein product as their main source of nutrition.

Regardless of their contents, most diets come and go, each enjoying a brief success. Some are funny and others phony.

Let's have a look at some of them.

The Harvard Diet (The cleverest.)
The Pizza Diet (The works.)
The Superstars' Diet (Not for everyone.)
The Cholesterol Diet (Your body produces the stuff anyway.)
The French Diet (Do they know something we don't?)
The Spinach Diet (For those who like fat forearms.)
The Glutton Diet (Doesn't work, believe me.)
The One-Pound-A-Day Diet (No more than six months.)
The Sacred Cow Diet (Very expensive importation.)
The Bread Lover's Diet (I know what's going on at the Bread Loaf Conference.)
The Busy Woman's Diet (*Apis lacris*—Latin name for honeybee.)
The Oriental Diet (Watch your eyes.)
The Beautiful Diet (Frankenstein, you go first.)
The Hot Days Diet (In winter you hibernate.)
The Negative Calories Diet (Really?)

The Cave Man's Diet (Brontosaurus steak only.)
The Free Diet (Who's gonna buy the food?)
The Cover Girl's Diet (I tried it once but my wife was jealous.)

Had enough? I was getting tired myself, and the list goes on and on—ad nauseam. More than half of these diets are a hoax; the rest of them are so dull they could make you cry uncle within a week.

With such diets your chance of losing weight and not putting it back are as good as playing Russian Roulette with five bullets in the cylinder without killing yourself!

Of course, a few diets are serious and effective, but most are complicated, impractical, and nutritionally ill-balanced. The most popular ones include Mayo, Stillman, Scarsdale, Pritikin, Beverly Hills, Atkins, and the Never-Say-Diet. Let's take the High-Protein-High-Fat Diet as an example. Excess protein in the body doesn't magically disappear. It is stored as fat. And an overconsumption of protein can produce too much uric acid in your body, which can lead to gout (arthritic attacks). As for high-fat consumption, it's completely irrational. With the caloric content of fat at *more than twice* the same quantity of carbohydrates or protein, your chances of losing weight are just about nil.

There is also the very popular High-Protein-Low-Carbohydrate Diet. Again, too much protein serves no useful purpose and low carbohydrates are a disaster. Carbohydrates are the main source of energy in your body. They also help metabolize fat. Your brain functions mainly on carbohydrates, so it's no wonder most people on low carb diets drag themselves around and feel grouchy. Natural carbohydrates are needed by your body in reasonable amounts. They are the real *energizers*.

Some diets idolatrize one food in particular—grapefruit, pineapple, eggs, fish, cottage cheese, steak, or (don't laugh) water. Proponents of such diets go as far as giving you a badge with the object of their reverence showing on it (provided you have eaten enough of the miraculous food, I suppose).

Finally, there are certain diets that get you to weigh every ounce of food you eat, to write down everything you eat during the week, how many burps you make at each meal, etc. Unless you are a zombie, you can't stick to such a diet for the rest of your life. Such behavior is not only compulsive, it's also ridiculous.

Here are Ten Golden Rules of a good diet.

1. A good diet is one you can follow year-round.
2. A good diet should be healthy—as healthy as you want to be.

3. A good diet should be versatile.
4. A good diet should be adaptable to eating out.
5. A good diet must include a large choice of foods to avoid boredom.
6. A good diet must permit you to indulge in your favorite dish once in a while to prevent a frustration buildup.
7. A good diet should keep your blood sugar normal so you're not always hungry.
8. A good diet must be simple: nothing to write down, nothing to weigh, no meetings and nothing fancy to buy except your regular groceries.
9. A good diet is one that becomes your life style.
10. A good diet should give you the feeling you are in control of it, not the other way around. In short, a good diet must make you happy.

As biased as it may sound, I do think that the Cheater's Diet offers you all of the above-mentioned and then some.

4

WHEN THREE MINUS TWO MAKES FAT

And gain is gain, however small. (Robert Browning)

Calories make you fat, right?

Wrong. Calories per se are not the problem. Only *an excess* of calories can make you fat. A huge excess of calories can get you fat in just a few days, while a small excess of calories can do the same over a period of many months. Much has been written about calories and I don't think there's anything new about it either. With the Cheater's Diet you will not have to count the exact number of calories you eat in a day, but having a rough idea of how much you take in should be your aim.

But first, what is a calorie?

Simply put, a calorie is a unit for measuring the amount of energy present in food. Food is the fuel that keeps your body bodying! No matter how you look at it, calories are the cornerstone of every diet. Don't let anyone kid you: *There's no way around it.* Any calorie *can* make you fat, whether it comes from fat, protein, or carbohydrates. For example, five hundred calories from chicken give the same energy as five hundred calories from butter. Both can make you fat if taken in excess. But to get five hundred calories from each, you would need to eat only five tablespoons of butter compared to three breasts of chicken.

All foods contain calories. Tea and coffee have none; but they are slow poisons rather than food. Water has no calories either, but it is essential to the maintenance of life. Vitamin pills have no calories, or only traces—nothing to worry about.

The three basic components of food are:

1. protein (lean meat, lean fish, egg white, etc.)
2. fats (butter, salad oil, cream, etc.)
3. carbohydrates (fruits, vegetables, bread, etc.)

Of those three, fats contain the most calories. Usually, fat has more than twice as many calories as either protein or carbohydrates. For example, one tablespoon of vegetable oil (fat) contains 120 calories while the same quantity of maple syrup (carbohydrates) has only fifty.

Foods containing mostly fat are extremely concentrated sources of calories and thus are easier to take in excess. To put it simply, an excess of fat makes you fat faster than an excess of protein or carbohydrates. Plain logic, isn't it?

THE FOOD SOURCE OF CALORIES DOES MATTER

Try this test at home: tomorrow morning. Eat a piece of chocolate cake for breakfast, and nothing else, except a few sips of water, if you feel like it. Then when you feel hungry again, take note of the time elapsed since your breakfast. The following morning, eat two boiled eggs and a banana. Again take note of how long it takes before you feel hungry.

The breakfasts suggested above contain approximately the same amount of calories, about two hundred and fifty. Yet, if you eat the chocolate cake, you'll feel hungry an hour or two later; however, eating the eggs and banana will get you through to lunch very easily. The reason is that most cake has less protein and fat than eggs, and bananas contain fiber. The digestion of protein and fat takes more time than that of carbohydrates, and fiber is hydrophilic—that is, fiber swells as it holds water and it causes distention in the stomach, thus creating a feeling of satiety.

Likewise, if you have cola and chips for lunch, your chances of making it to dinner without eating again are slim, and if you do, you'll be so hungry by then that you will overeat. On the other hand, if you have two bananas and a glass of skim milk for lunch you can make it to dinner without going on a binge. Of course, this example applies more to an office worker than to a six-foot-three lumberjack. Your caloric intake should be determined by your age, weight, height, sex, and, above all, by your metabolism and the type of work you do. This means that you can get fat on 2,000 calories a day while someone else will be lean on 4,000 a day. Among the biggest eaters in the world are the boatmen of the Rhine, who average 5,200 calories daily.

In 1976 at the Montreal Olympic Games, a survey was conducted among the athletes to find the main factor in superior athletic performance. The answer was calories—a *lot* of calories. The study indicated that Olympic athletes averaged between 4,000 and 6,000 calories a day and most of them attributed their superior performance to the energy produced by such a large caloric intake. Watching the games on television, you may have noticed the absence of fat on their bodies. I see two reasons for this: They train intensively every day for long hours and, like most athletes, they have a fast or medium metabolism.

Of course, there are exceptions among athletes—for example, Vassili Alexeiev, the Russian weightlifter. At six-foot-one and 330 pounds he's not exactly lean, but he is a phenomenon. What else would you call someone who eats a two-dozen-egg omelette and a whole chicken at one sitting and washes it down with two quarts of milk?

HOW AN EXCESS OF CALORIES MAKES YOU FAT

Let's say you weigh 150 pounds and need 2,000 calories a day to maintain your normal body weight, and suppose that your three meals a day add up to the required 2,000 calories. That's what we call your maintenance level (caloric intake).

What would happen if every night, besides your regular meals, you ate a chocolate sundae containing 1,000 calories? This would increase your daily caloric intake from 2,000 to 3,000. You'd be 1,000 calories over your requirement, and if you did this for a week, you would be 7,000 calories over. We know that a pound of fat is equal to 3,500 calories, so if you divide 7,000 by 3,500 you have a gain of two pounds of fat in one week.

Let's say this gain of two pounds of fat frightened you and you went back to about 2,000 calories a day, would you lose the two pounds you had gained? No, because 2,000 calories is your maintenance level. So if you want to lose weight, you have to eat fewer calories—a *lot* less than your maintenance level. If you drop your caloric intake to 1,000 a day, you would be 1,000 short of your maintenance level and at the end of a week you would lose 7,000 calories or two pounds.

In short, to gain a pound of fat, you must eat 3,500 calories more than your body needs and to lose the same pound of fat you have to eat 3,500 calories less than your body needs, regardless of the time span involved.

That's as much as you have to know about calories. This and the fact that all fats contain *more than twice* as many calories as an equal amount of protein or carbohydrates.

Next you'll find a calorie chart of the most common foods. Study it carefully.

Note: You may find slight variations in the caloric value of some foods from one calorie chart to another. For example, the calorie value of one tablespoon of honey is relatively stable; however, trying to establish the precise caloric value of a piece of apple pie or a slice of pizza is a little tricky. Many factors can influence the caloric computing of foods, such as the amount of different ingredients in its composition, the size of the serving, the way it's cooked, etc.

Overall, however, we can safely say that the calorie chart below is as close to reality as possible.

CALORIE CHART OF THE MOST COMMON FOODS

Foods	*Measure*	*Calories*
Almonds, unsalted	10 to 12	72
Apple	1 medium	80
Apple juice, canned	4 oz.	58
Apricot juice	4 oz.	72
Applesauce, sweetened	4 oz.	116
Applesauce, unsweetened	4 oz.	50
Apricots	1 medium	20
Apricots, canned	½ cup	110
Asparagus	8 spears (fresh and cooked)	24
Avocado, raw	½ medium	200
Bacon: crisp, fried	2 slices	90
Banana	1 medium	95
Beef (hamburger), uncooked	4 oz.	235
Beef (sirloin steak), broiled	4 oz.	432
Beef liver, fried	4 oz.	260
Beets, cooked, diced	½ cup	20
Beer	8 ounces	101
Blueberries, fresh	½ cup	45
Bread (whole wheat)	1 slice	68
Bread (white)	1 slice	70
Bread (pumpernickel)	1 slice	78
Bread (rye)	1 slice	60
Bread crumbs: fresh, unbuttered	½ cup	62
Broccoli, cooked	½ cup	20
Brussels sprouts, cooked	1 cup	56
Buckwheat: whole, raw	¾ cup	335

Foods	Measure	Calories
Butter	4 tablespoons	400
Buttermilk	4 oz.	44
Cabbage: green, boiled	½ cup	15
Cantaloupe	one half	60
Carrots: raw	1 large	30
Carrots, cooked	½ cup, diced	22
Cashew nuts	4	46
Cauliflower, cooked	½ cup	14
Celery, raw	1 stalk	8
Cereal (oatmeal)	4 oz. (cooked)	63
Cereal (shredded wheat)	1 biscuit	89
Cereal (whole wheat)	½ cup	54
Cheese (cheddar)	4 oz.	452
Cheese (cottage—low fat)	½ cup	90
Chicken, skinned	1 breast (cooked)	166
Chocolate	4 oz. (sweet)	600
Chocolate cake	1 slice (medium)	365
Clams, canned	½ cup	52
Coconut, dried	1 oz. (shredded)	187
Cola drinks	8 ounces	96
Cookies (chocolate chip)	1	50
Corn, whole kernel	½ cup (canned)	87
Corn, cream style	½ cup	105
Cream	4 tablespoons	212
Cucumber	6 slices	5
Dates, dried/pitted	½ cup	270
Doughnuts (jelly-filled)	1	226
Eggs, poached	1 large	82
Figs (dried)	1 large	60
Fish (haddock)	4 oz. (fried)	188
Fish (salmon)	4 oz. (broiled)	208
Fish (tuna)	½ cup (canned in oil)	158
Fish (tuna)	½ cup (canned in water)	126
Flour (all-purpose)	1 cup, sifted	420
Flour (whole wheat)	1 cup, sifted	400

Foods	Measure	Calories
Garlic, peeled	1 clove	4
Grapefruit (white)	1 medium	112
Grapefruit (pink)	1 medium	116
Grapes: green, fresh	½ cup	48
Grapes: concord, fresh	½ cup	35
Ham	4 oz. (cooked)	496
Honey	1 tablespoon	64
Ice cream, vanilla	½ cup	320
Ice cream, chocolate	½ cup	400
Ice milk	1 cup	199
Jam	1 tablespoon	54
Lamb, loin chop/lean	4 oz.	215
Lima beans, fresh	½ cup	95
Lime	1 medium	19
Lemon	1 medium	20
Lobster, cooked meat	3 ounces	80
Macaroni	1 cup (cooked)	190
Maple syrup	1 tablespoon	50
Margarine	4 tablespoons	400
Mayonnaise	4 tablespoons	360
Milk (regular)	1 cup	159
Milk (skim)	1 cup	88
Milk (evaporated)	1 cup	172
Molasses	1 tablespoon	50
Muffins (bran)	1	104
Mushrooms	4 large	28
Mustard	2 tablespoons	24
Noodles	1 cup (cooked)	200
Oil (all kinds)	1 tablespoon	120
Olives	6 medium	23
Onion, raw	1 medium	40
Orange	1 medium	64
Oysters	½ cup (raw)	80
Papaya	1 small	43

Foods	Measure	Calories
Parsley	5 tablespoons	5
Pancakes	1 (4-inch diameter)	61
Peaches	1 medium	38
Peanut butter	4 tablespoons	380
Pears	1 medium	100
Peas, fresh	½ cup (cooked)	57
Peppers, green, raw	1 medium	16
Pineapple, fresh	½ cup	40
Pizza	1 slice (average)	153
Plum, fresh	1 medium	25
Pork, loin chop, lean	4 ounces	280
Potatoes	1 medium (raw or baked)	86
Radishes, raw	10 small	10
Rice (white)	½ cup (cooked)	112
Rice (brown)	½ cup (cooked)	116
Salad dressing		
(French)	1 tablespoon	66
(Italian)	1 tablespoon	83
Sauerkraut, canned	½ cup	20
Shrimp, canned	4 ounces (cooked)	140
Spaghetti	1 cup (cooked)	172
Spinach	1 cup (canned)	44
Strawberries	½ cup (fresh)	28
Sugar (brown)	1 tablespoon	50
Tangerine	1 medium	40
Tea		0
Tomatoes, fresh	1 medium	27
Turkey, roast	4 ounces	214
Veal, cooked, cutlet	4 ounces	230
Vinegar	1 tablespoon	2
Wheat germ	1 tablespoon	23
Yogurt, plain, skim milk	½ cup	61
Zucchini	½ cup (cooked)	16
Zwieback	1 cracker	30

5

HOW MUCH IS "NOT MUCH"?

Whatever you cannot understand, you cannot possess. (Johann Wolfgang von Goethe)

I'm sure Einstein wasn't preoccupied with such a trivial matter as losing weight when he returned home from a walk and wrote his famous equation, $E = Mc^2$. Yet many things in life are relative, even in the shape-up game, as we'll see now.

Many years ago (before I had formulated the Cheater's Diet) when I advised my gym's members on dieting, I would simply tell them to eat less—to stay hungry if they wanted to lose weight. Usually, this practice coupled with a rigorous exercise program did the trick. Yet one of my woman customers complained that she couldn't lose a single pound, despite the fact that she was not eating much. To find out how much was "not much," I asked her to write down what she had eaten that day. For her, a light breakfast was a bowl of hot oatmeal with milk and sugar, three pieces of toast with jam and cheese, and a small glass of milk. "Not much" was actually about eight or nine hundred calories. This may have been okay if she had been a marathoner but she was a secretary sitting at a desk all day. At five-foot-three and one hundred and twenty-five pounds, she was lucky to have maintained her body weight despite such eating habits. I advised her to skip the glass of milk and to have only one piece of toast without any cheese. Within a month, the delighted woman had lost six pounds.

This incident reminds me of a test done in a hospital among obese patients. They were weighed, then asked how much they thought they ate. As you may have guessed, the answer was "not much." Then each patient was asked to write down the amount of food he or she ingested in one day, and for the next two weeks each was fed exactly what he or she had indicated. At the end of the test, they were all weighed again and *all* had lost a significant amount of weight.

KEEP YOUR INDIVIDUALITY IN SIGHT

The story (fiction) goes like this:

Jenny wakes up one morning and rolls her flabby 160-pound body out of bed. She looks in the mirror and feels disgusted. Then she remembers what she read the day before in the *Hollywood Gazette* about her favorite movie star who lost ten pounds with the Cheater's Diet and looked gorgeous in her yellow bikini. Summer is only a few months away and Jenny decides that this year she's going to have her share of beach parties. So she rushes out to the book store and buys a copy of *The Cheater's Diet*. Jenny figures that losing 40 pounds by the summer should make her look just like her movie star idol. After four months on the Cheater's Diet, Jenny has made it. She now weighs a hundred and twenty pounds. Yet somehow there's a great difference between what she sees in the mirror and her idol's picture. Jenny will probably live with a bittersweet feeling for a while.

This story was not meant to discourage you but to warn you against setting your goals too high and losing sight of your own individuality.

Each of us is unique. No two persons have the same muscle and bone density. For example, two persons have the same height and weight. Why is it that one of them can float easily in water while the other will sink like a rock? The same thing applies with appearances. A few years ago I was competing in the World Wristwrestling Championship. I made my way to the finals and ended up against the defending champion—a really skinny guy, the same height as I was. He beat me. After the match, many people asked me how a scrawny guy like that could beat me. They all said I looked 25 to 30 pounds heavier than he did. I had no answer until I asked him to jump on the scale—he weighed three pounds more than I did.

So take stock of your unique self and be realistic. If you're a woman and you were born with wide hips, nothing will make them narrower. If you're a man and you were born with narrow shoulders, nothing will make them wider. But that doesn't mean you are out of the running just because you don't have it all. Make the best of what you have; at least you can be healthy, fit, and better looking.

WEIGHT LOSS VS. FAT LOSS

Weight loss doesn't always indicate fat loss. Your body is made of about seventy percent water and through perspiration you lose a surprising amount of fluid. For women, menstruation is a factor that can negatively influence their body weight.

Women should wait until after their period to weigh themselves. And whether you're a man or a woman, your body weight can be affected by a bout with the flu but it won't be a fat loss, just a temporary water loss (dehydration). Be aware of your body fluctuations and don't conclude instantly that you've gained or lost weight. Wait three days and weigh yourself again before making any adjustments in your diet.

So beware of elusive weight loss. Make sure your weight loss is a *fat* loss; computers are getting better and better but technicians have yet to come up with a talking scale that tells you the facts about your body weight fluctuations.

APPETITE AND HUNGER

There's a subtle difference between these two: appetite is the desire (psychological) for certain foods while hunger is a strong need (physical) for any kind of food. What you eat can have a lot to do with the control you have over appetite and hunger. Refined sugar (simple carbohydrates) gets into your bloodstream relatively fast but it doesn't satisfy you for long because it lacks nutrients. On the other hand, the assimilation of a meal composed of complex carbohydrates (bread, potato, cereal) and protein will be slower (especially the protein) and the satisfaction you derive from such a meal will last much longer. If you eat as indicated in the Cheater's Diet, you won't be bothered with false appetite; the hunger you'll experience will be derived from a real physiological need.

HOW TO READ FOOD LABELS

Most of the foods we buy at the supermarket have labels listing their ingredients. Of course, fruit, meat, and eggs have no labels because we all know what they are made of. Or do we?

Food manufacturers who do not label their products or who label them dishonestly are infringing on one of our basic rights—the right to be informed.

The ingredients on a food label are listed in order of importance: The first listed ingredient is the one of greatest quantity in the product. For example, a cereal box label says: sugar, puffed rice, honey, BTH. This means the major ingredient in the box is sugar, followed closely (how closely, we don't know) by puffed rice, and then some honey and a small amount of BTH—probably enough to keep the box on the shelf six months longer than it should be.

How Much Is "Not Much"?

Sometimes reading labels can be tricky. Take the case of whole wheat bread, for example. You have decided to eat nothing but 100 percent whole wheat and you rush to the supermarket to buy the "real thing." All you have to do is make sure that "100% whole wheat bread" is written on the package. Right? Wrong—completely wrong. There is real whole wheat bread and there's phony whole wheat bread. Complicated? Not really. Let's read the label of phony wheat bread.

100% Whole Wheat Bread

Ingredients: Whole wheat flour, sugar and/or liquid sugar and/or glucose-fructose and/or dextrose, vegetable oil shortening (may contain palm oil), salt, extra fancy molasses, yeast, wheat gluten, calcium sulfate, ammonium chloride, potassium bromate, calcium propinate, may contain protease and/or calcium peroxide.

Phony enough for you? Why don't they know from day to day what they're going to put in their so-called whole wheat bread? Why would one swallow potassium bromate? To lessen one's sexual drive maybe? And what about this sulfate, chloride, and peroxide? To bleach your guts perhaps? Why those poisons in your bread? To make more money and/or to keep the product on the shelf longer and/or to make people think they are buying whole wheat bread when actually they are buying white bread coloured with extra fancy molasses and/or caramel.

Now here's how a *real* 100% whole wheat bread label should read:

Ingredients: Whole wheat flour, water, sunflower oil, pure cane sugar, sea salt, yeast.

That's a simple label, isn't it? And the bread is better tasting too. Also the wrapping on the real whole wheat loaf often carries a warning to keep the bread refrigerated for better conservation, plus some information that reads like this:

Weight per slice	34.8 g
H_2O	15.0 g
Ashes	77.0 g
Proteins	4.0 g
Carbohydrates	20.0 g
Calories per slice	68

In short, the more information on the label and the wrapping on how the product is made, the better it is. Bread manufacturers should mention if their flour is stone-ground, whether they use spring water, and other relevant details you are entitled to know. If you're allergic to sulfate and the label says the product may or may not have sulfate, what do you do? Take a chance and end up in the hospital? Or, if your doctor has told you to avoid salt and the product says it may or may not contain salt, what do you do? Boycott any food product whose label says it may or may not contain this or that ingredient. You have a right to know what you're putting into your body.

6

BEWARE OF RIP-OFFS

The prudence of the best heads is often defeated by the tenderness of the best hearts. (Henry Fielding)

So many rip-offs center on fatness today that I thought you ought to know of at least a few of the common ones and why they are rip-offs. In case you were contemplating the idea of investing some money in one of them, read this first.

SAUNA

Sauna is defined in the dictionary as a steam bath treatment but there's no mention as to *what* is treated. Maybe they will find something to treat in the future with the sauna. Meanwhile at the OK Corral, ranch people are using the sauna hoping to shed fat. Paying a few dollars to take a sauna in a spa is one thing, but if you're buying a $1,000 sauna to put in your basement because the salesman convinced you it's the best way to lose fat, that's a big rip-off.

Let's say you've been in a sauna for half an hour to one hour. You get out and jump on the scale. Bingo, two pounds less. How easy. At that rate you would have lost up to 48 pounds in a day. Great. The problem is, however, that what you've lost is not two pounds of fat but two pounds of water, for your body is about *70 percent* water. So as soon as you have a few glasses of water and an "oh-so-very-light meal," you will be back at the starting gate again. You will have regained two pounds.

You can't lose fat in a sauna because you are sitting idle on a bench staring at the wall. You are not using any calories in the form of energy. It's as if you were sitting in front of the TV at home on a hot and humid summer day, nothing more.

The only thing a sauna can do for you is help you relax and clean the pores of your skin and this is not without side effects. If you stay in too long (20 minutes and up) you can experience dizziness, nosebleeds, and the like. Moreover, if you go to a sauna on a daily basis, you can end up with burns of the respiratory tract tissues. The Finns, who use a sauna extensively (they invented it), suffer from this condition (which is a form of cancer) more than anyone else. So take this into account before you take a sauna bath, let alone buy one. And a final point: Frequent sauna sessions can *lower* the production of sperm cells in males.

MASSAGE

If I became a rich man, I would hire a geisha girl and make sure I had my daily massage. I love the feeling of a good massage. In addition it helps to relax one's muscles and improve blood circulation. But (at twenty dollars an hour) if someone told you massages are going to get rid of unwanted fat, it *is* a rip-off. As in the sauna, you're lying idle while the masseuse is working on you. She's the one who's burning calories, not you. It's a fact, however, that a deep massage can produce involuntary contractions of muscles; that's why you may be sore the day after. But the amount of work thus generated (calories burned) is trifling, to say the least. Enjoy a good massage but never rely on this practice to lose unwanted fat.

BODY WRAP

"Lose between 3 and 6 inches in an hour at home" reads the advertisement. Sauna suits and various body wraps are common rip-offs. These gadgets work on the same principle as the steam bath. The idea is to get enough heat around the body, or a specific part of the body, to temporarily dehydrate it. So if there's any reduction, it's due only to water loss, not fat loss.

Have you noticed when you buy one of these suits or wraps that the manufacturer always recommends you exercise while wearing the gadget? The analogy that can be made here is with the cereal manufacturer who claims his product is a good source of protein—when you add six ounces of milk to it, that is.

NATURAL FAT EMULSIFIER AND DIURETIC

"Melt the fat away—only three capsules before meals—lose up to 25 pounds in a week." Some health food manufacturers try to sell a combopack of different natural products designed to emulsify human fat. The most common formula is apple cider vinegar, kelp, vitamin B6 and lecithin; the formula *doesn't work*. Even the most vigorous exercise is not a fat emulsifier. The only way to burn fat in your body is to create a caloric deficiency; in this way your stored fat is used as a source of energy. The same thing applies to the other well-known combination of choline and inositol (sometimes classified as B complex vitamin). I know a guy who has been taking massive doses of these two products for several years and he's still fat. A meal for him consists invariably of a soup, a main dish with bread and a dessert. I finally talked him into skipping the soup, bread, and dessert but, unfortunately, he's still wasting his money on choline and inositol.

Another rip-off is that vitamin C taken in large amounts, two grams and more a day, will act as a natural diuretic. A diuretic is a product that tends to increase the discharge of urine. But two grams of vitamin C can have a drug-like effect on your body. Moreover, you don't urinate fat, you burn it by using it as energy.

CREAMS AND LOTIONS

If you believe in the Jesus Christ Diet (you pray the fat away—no joke), if you believe in the Cold Water Diet (ten glasses of cold water a day to dilute fat), if you believe that love at first sight is commonplace, then you are a potential client for the numerous creams and lotions advertised as thigh, waist, and bottom slimmers. These creams do *absolutely nothing* —no more than the creams that guarantee flat-chested women they will put four inches on the bust within two weeks.

If you've used such creams or lotions you might have been fooled by the tingling effect on your skin after you applied it. That feeling wasn't caused by an enzyme eating the fat away; it was just a chemical in the cream that triggers a placebo effect in your mind—amen.

STARCH BLOCKERS

If you like potatoes, pasta, and bread but you want to lose weight, you need . . . Starch Blockers? No. All you need are facts. First, there's absolutely nothing wrong with starches like potatoes or whole wheat bread. Your body can efficiently use the wholesome nutrients they provide: vitamins, minerals, and fiber. The only starches you must be leary of are pasta. Don't eat pasta on a regular basis (only on your cheating meals) because it is so refined that (nutritionally speaking) it cannot sustain you for long.

Starches, carbohydrates, and fats per se don't make you fat; an *excess* of them makes you fat. Fatty foods are higher in calories and studies show that the average American gets 70 percent of his total caloric intake from fat. That's where the problem comes from.

Instead of reducing their fat intake, most people look for the easy way out. They will try any new product without weighing the implications, without searching for the soundness behind the idea and foreseeing the possible long-term effects on their health.

Basically, Starch Blockers are made from protein extract found in raw kidney beans. Starch Blockers interfere with the action of the enzymes that digests starch. So the starch is eliminated from the body unused; or so goes the theory. The problem with Starch Blockers is that manufacturers would like people to believe they can eat all the starch they want and still not gain weight. But this isn't so. Their weight loss plan allows for only 700 starch calories daily. No smorgasborgs or fiestas obviously. Suppose you're a French fries addict, you can burn only 400 hundred calories of starch (potatoes) with one pill. But most of the calories in French fries come from the oil in which they are fried. Not much help, as you can see. Same thing for a pizza maniac who plans to use Starch Blockers—the calories in a pizza come mostly from the oil, cheese, meat, and gravy, not the flour.

As for the side effects of Starch Blockers, they may include interference in protein digestion, abnormal clotting of the blood, allergic reactions to kidney beans, and diarrhea. If you feel no side effects you are probably paying for a placebo.

If Starch Blockers are such a big sell-out, it only proves how naive people can be sometimes.

7

SHATTERING A FEW MYTHS

Nothing is so firmly believed as that which we least know. (Michel de Montaigne)

Of all the people I've seen fighting and losing the battle of the bulge over the years, I've noticed they all lacked willpower or knowledge, or both. Willpower is mainly subjective; it has to do with how badly you want to reach your goal. As for knowledge, part of it depends on your educational background and part on your intellectual curiosity. Yet myths die hard and many well-educated people not only believe in those dietary myths but spread them around with religious zeal.

Let's take a look at the most common dietary myths.

BREAD

Invariably, when someone proudly announces that he's going on a diet, he will say something about cutting out bread from his diet, vaguely mentioning that bread is fattening because it has so many calories. But a slice of bread has an average of only 68 calories compared with a medium-sized apple, which has eighty. Granted it's easier to eat five slices of bread in a row than five apples and most people put butter on their bread, but who says you have to put butter on your toast and eat five slices per sitting? Instead, it's better to put one tablespoon of honey on your toast for breakfast or take two slices and make yourself a delicious banana sandwich that would only yield about 200 calories. As you can see, there would be room enough for more calories to make an interesting meal. In the Cheater's Diet, if you like bread, you eat bread because it's not a concentrated source of calories like butter. I'm referring to 100 percent whole wheat bread not white bread, which is not a food as far as I'm concerned. White bread makes you constipated because it has no fiber. Try this simple test: Take a slice of whole wheat and try to make a ball out of it with your hands. You can't because wheat fiber won't stick together. Now try to do the same thing with a slice of white bread. You'll get a round puttylike ball that sticks together because it has no fiber and is full of chemicals. The choice is yours.

POTATOES

Potatoes are about as mythical as bread for the average dieter. Again the same old song: it's fattening—too many calories. Yet one look at a calorie chart will show you that a medium-sized potato has 86 calories, only six calories more than an apple. So why the fuss? Again the answer lies in the preparation of the food. Potatoes are mashed, then milk is added (for consistency) and butter (for flavor). Some people even add eggs to make the whole thing stickier, but milk and eggs don't add any flavor to potatoes, they add only calories.

Boiled in water without salt, potatoes are OK. If it's flavor and nutrition you want, bake it with the skin. A potato contains vitamins A, B, C, calcium, phosphorus, iron, protein, and complex carbohydrates (a good source of sustained-release energy). Indeed, the potato is one of the best foods to include in your Cheater's Diet menu.

BANANA

The banana may not be as taboo as bread and potatoes in most dieters' minds but it's still a no-no in order to lose weight, regardless of the fact that a banana has only 95 calories. And bananas have vitamins A, B, C, calcium, potassium and are a good source of natural carbohydrates. So as a dieter, bananas are excellent for you, unless you eat them daily as part of a banana-split sundae. As a bonus, the banana has antacid properties and is one of the easiest foods to digest.

GRAPEFRUIT

Now here's the biggest joke of them all. I don't remember who started the rumor, but one day every dieter seemed to be praising the virtues of grapefruit as a fat burner. Wouldn't it be nice if it were true? Unfortunately, no food can claim the title of "fat burner," all foods contain calories and any food eaten in excess can make you fat. Speaking of calories, a cup of grapefruit juice has 101 calories compared to 112 for a cup of orange juice. Now suppose you are at your normal body weight and you're eating about the right number of calories to keep it that way, what would happen if you started to drink two cups of grapefruit juice every day, along with your regular meals and beverages? Theoretically, 35 days later you would be two pounds heavier because you would have gained an excess of 7,000 calories. That's all you need know about grapefruit, which is, nonetheless, an excellent food.

PINEAPPLE

Pineapple is one of my favorite fruits; however, I don't believe its enzymes can eat away body fat like hungry piranha fish. Yet pineapple seems to have replaced grapefruit lately as the fat burner par excellence! There's no scientific basis to back up this theory, and like any other food, pineapple eaten in excess can make you fat.

CHOLESTEROL AND EGGS

The cholesterol craze started in 1913 when a Russian scientist showed that feeding cholesterol to rabbits induced heart diseases. But because rabbits are vegetarians, their systems cannot handle cholesterol from an animal source. There is no conclusive proof showing that eating eggs increases the risk of heart attack among healthy people.

Consider the following facts:

1. Your body produces cholesterol every day.
2. When you cut down on cholesterol in your diet, your body tends to produce more of it to compensate for the reduced intake.

Maybe nature is trying to tell us something. However, a noted physician stated that cholesterol-related problems are individual in nature. Just as diabetics have problems with sugar, others have problems with cholesterol.

The American physician J. I. Rodale ate 36 egg yolks daily for three months without any increase in his cholesterol count. I've always been fond of eggs. A few years ago, I ate *sixteen* eggs a day for many months in an effort to gain strength for a wristwrestling competition. I also had my cholesterol checked at the hospital while on this massive egg intake and it was normal. Today I still eat from one to two dozen eggs a week and my cholesterol count is right where it should be.

If you're an office worker spending your evenings in front of the tube and you eat two dozen eggs a day, you might be inviting problems. Ditto if you eat 24 bananas a day. Even water in excess is not good for your system.

Eggs are one of the most perfect foods: inexpensive, easy to digest, unprocessed, and high in protein. Egg yolk contains a great deal of lecithin, which plays an important role in fat metabolism. Yet sedentary people who wouldn't touch an egg with a ten-foot pole think nothing of putting large amounts of butter on their vegetables, or eating French fries, or putting cream in their coffee. What's the logic of that behavior?

The problem is not the eggs; it's not even the cholesterol; it's our whole way of life. Smoking, eating junk foods, little or no exercise, pollution, and stress are responsible for more heart attacks than all the eggs in the world.

BUTTER VS. MARGARINE

The myth is that margarine is better for you than butter, but better for what? Certainly not for losing weight because margarine has the same caloric content as butter. Both should not be taken regularly because they are concentrated sources of calories.

Dietetic considerations aside, butter is natural, since it's made from cream. On the other hand, margarine is computer-made and anything can enter its fabrication. Ask yourself why margarine doesn't require refrigeration while butter does.

THE FAT-CELL THEORY

There are many theories on obesity. Not all fat people are responsible for their misfortune, and these theories are actually excuses to enjoy plumpness without guilt. Supposedly, many obese people are overweight because they lack an enzyme found in red blood cells. If that were true, why is it that this phenomenon is found in overabundant societies *only*? Why is it that people in the Third World are not suffering from obesity? The reason: not a lack of enzymes but a lack of calories.

Another myth is that once you get fat your body retains a memory of those fat cells and you will always be fighting your body momentum toward obesity. *Ridiculous!* Being obese is not a natural condition and when you're slim again your body momentum will tend toward a well-balanced condition. You and *only you* can reverse that momentum by forced-feeding on junk foods.

The same is true for a skinny person who returned to his normal body weight. His body momentum would tend to keep his normal weight stable and not to make him skinny again. In the gym business, I've seen hundreds of men and women lose fat and reach their normal weight; yet each time some of them become fat again. But it was not because they had come under the influence of their body momentum; it was because they had started to "pig-out" again, which they openly admitted.

8

IN CASE YOU ASK

No man really becomes a fool until he stops asking questions. (Charles Steinmetz)

THE CHEATER'S DIET—QUESTIONS AND ANSWERS

How long will it take with the Cheater's Diet to reach my ideal weight?

Between two weeks and six months or more, depending on how fat you are to begin with and how seriously you apply the principles in this book. Compared to the time it took you to put on weight, the time it'll take to lose weight will be relatively short. The Cheater's Diet will not perform miracles. It's a way of life for intelligent people who want to lose fat (forever) and build up their health at the same time.

What is the only sweetener allowed in the regular part of the Cheater's Diet?

Unpasteurized honey. Unlike other forms of sugar (corn syrup, maple syrup, white sugar, fancy molasses), honey is not processed. It contains only small amounts of minerals and vitamins but it leaves an alkaline deposit in the body, which is desirable. The darker the honey, the more alkaline it is. Pasteurization is unnecessary for honey because it contains a natural preservative: formic acid. Honey was found in the Egyptian Pyramids and it was still edible. It should be used sparingly, however, more like a seasoning than a food because it is a concentrated source of calories. (A teaspoonful to a tablespoonful in yogurt, cereal, or on a piece of toast can put a smile back on your face while you are losing fat.) Speaking of sugar, blackstrap molasses, although a sugar, doesn't taste sweet and should be considered as a food supplement. (For details on supplements, see Chapter 30.)

Is it true that if I eat only one kind of food at mealtime I will eat less of it?

How much you will eat of a particular food depends mainly on the texture of the food. It has nothing to do with how many kinds of food you eat at one sitting. Imagine yourself in front of the TV with a quart of ice cream and see how fast you can do away with it. On the other hand, how many raw carrots can you eat before you get tired of chewing? Not many. You will likely eat more pudding, jello, mousses, and whipped cream than chicken, nuts, and raw vegetables.

Is it advisable to lose weight fast?

No, especially if you are over thirty, obese, and don't exercise. Losing weight fast could be a stress on your heart and you may end up with so much loose skin around your body that you'll need surgery.

What's the first and foremost requirement of an effective diet?

Basically, it must be low in calories. *There's no way around it*, as scientific evidence shows.

Can you be fat yet, at the same time, be healthy and fit?

As long as you're not extremely fat, you can be overweight but healthy and fit, especially if you don't drink or smoke and have been exercising since your youth. Many retired athletes (but still active) are living proof of that. Their blood pressure and heart beat are normal, and they can do sommersaults and run a few miles. In short, they can outperform the average individual. But as a rule, too much fat is not a sign of health.

Is there a best time to start dieting?

Yes—when your mind has accepted the fact that you'll have to diet for *most* of your life and you *really* want to do so. In other words, a few days after you've finished reading *The Cheater's Diet*, when you're really psyched up.

I'm always craving sweets. How can I get rid of my obsession?

First, stop eating refined sugar and foods that contain it. You have an addiction to sugar. If your need for sugar persists two weeks after you have cut down on it, increase your protein intake; it is obviously too low.

Would it be better for an obese teenager to wait until he or she has matured physically before going on a diet?

Being young is no excuse for being fat. In fact, obesity can actually impair the sound development of a teenager, without mentioning the social hang-ups that may result at this critical time in life. Young people should follow a well-balanced diet, and taking natural food supplements would be a good idea at this stage of their life, considering their habit of skipping meals and their overindulgence in junk foods at times.

Should I rely on the conventional height-weight chart to determine my ideal weight?

Absolutely not; it's the worst thing you could do. Since everybody is so different, such charts are worthless.

What about food combinations? Are they of any importance for a dieter?

There is only one food combination that you should avoid on a daily basis and that's combining one junk food with another junk food. Why? Because they add up. An occasional meal made up of junk foods cannot hurt you because your body has the ability to detoxify itself of small amounts of poison. As for combining regular foods (for example, protein with carbs, carbs with vegetables, etc.), this theory doesn't hold water. Do you think that animals in their natural habitat worry about food combinations? Yet they are immune to cancer, heart disease, and the like, and they don't know heartburn, headaches, and flatulence; they eat whatever they want in no particular order or combinations. How many centenarians do you know who worry about making the "right" food combinations? I don't think you reach 100 by worrying at all—certainly not about food combinations.

What's so different about the Cheater's Diet?

It's a diet you can be proud of because it doesn't set you apart from the non-dieter. Yet your way of eating is ten times healthier. Your body can't get tired of the Cheater's Diet and your mind will thrive on it because it's the most exciting and versatile diet ever conceived. Anyone, anywhere, anytime, and for as long as he or she wants, can live by the philosophy of the Cheater's Diet. Since you will cheat sometimes anyway, why not plan it and enjoy it if you can lose fat in the process? Cheating everyday on your diet, as the non-dieter does, can be boring, but cheating every four days makes for a much-awaited meal. That's where you have an advantage over non-dieters while you look forward to reaching your desired weight.

I take all my vitamin pills (A, B, C, D, E) after my breakfast. A friend of mine told me that's not a good idea because the vitamins cancel each other when taken together. For example, vitamin E cancels vitamin C. Is this true?

It's not true. Vitamins almost always occur together in natural foods because they work together.

What form of exercise would best complement the Cheater's Diet?

Body building—definitely. Not because it burns more calories than other forms but because body building has a cosmetic effect on your shape. From a dieter's point of view, no other exercise works the body so completely. Also, a good body building program can create an illusion of slimness in body parts that are genetically too well-endowed to ever look thin with regular exercise. Example: A woman who has a big hip structure can create an illusion of slimness in her lower body by reducing the sides of her thighs and building up the muscles located on the side of the waist, just above the hip bone. Likewise a man who has a naturally broad waist structure can make it appear smaller by building up the lateral deltoids (the muscles on the side of the shoulder). Also, body building can be done year-round, since it's done inside, and you can choose the day and hours you want to train. Indeed, body building is the perfect activity for all dieters: it gives you good muscle tone, tightens skin, improves your posture, and boosts your confidence. It gives you the look of a winner.

Is it true that if I eat only one food at mealtime, it will be so completely digested that I can eat as much as I want without getting fat?

You be the judge. Try this: Eat a small jar of peanut butter at each meal for a week—and nothing else but water. If you haven't gained weight at the end of that week, write to the *Guinness Book of Records* because you just set a record. Your body doesn't differentiate between calories from a single-food meal and a multiple-food meal. If you eat too many calories, you'll gain weight. On the other hand, Eskimos eat single-food meals that are very high in fats and they are not exactly skinny people.

Some nutrition experts believe that all juices should be banned from a diet. Is there anything wrong with juices?

This belief comes from a purist theory that juice lacks fiber, thus making it an incomplete food. The importance of fiber, however, has been overrated recently. Fiber doesn't *feed* you. Calories do. If you had to choose between eggs (no fiber) and celery (high fiber) as your unique source of nourishment for the next three months, which one would you pick? Juices (unsweetened and in small amounts, of course) are good for dieters, although some of them are too high in calories to be included in the Cheater's Diet. Banning all juices from a diet is like trying to be more religious than the Pope. In the hot summer months a glass of juice on the rocks is like a cool breeze.

Why do most diets fail in the long run?

Because they are either boring or they leave you no energy to do anything else besides dieting. Most diets are conceived on paper first as fancy theories and are tested later with the public as guinea pigs. But they can't be followed continuously because too much emphasis is put on the technical side of losing weight and not enough on the life-style of the dieter. In addition to being basically low in calories, a permanent diet must allow you to indulge occasionally in your favorite foods in a controlled manner.

Part II

Who Are You?

9

THE DIETER'S PROFILE

Everyone is a moon, and has a dark side which he never shows to anybody.
(Mark Twain)

Your dieting profile, or the way you eat on a daily basis, has more psychological than physical implications. Once you understand the reasons behind your behavioral eating patterns, you can progressively work them out with such tools as self-hypnosis, motivation techniques, and avoidance of no-contest situations until you reach a healthier eating scheme.

Generally speaking, the eating profiles of fat people show a common trait. When these people suffer a setback of any kind or when they are emotionally upset, they go on eating binges. The amount of food consumed at such times is usually proportional to the severity of the disturbance. In overeating they are trying to compensate for their frustrations, only to be confronted with another one—that of getting fatter. And whatever they may say to the contrary, fat people don't like being fat. Again frustrated, they eat more; it is a vicious circle that must be broken to get weight back to normal and keep it stable. The reasons for such behavior are often affective in nature and are probably deeply rooted in one's childhood. But it is not in the domain of a diet book to make an in-depth study of such motivations. In the next chapters, however, we will explore six of the most common profiles in eating behavior and give hints on how to break free of them.

BODY TYPES

A physical aspect that may be related to an eating profile is body type. Basically there are three body types: ectomorph, mesomorph, and endomorph. Few people belong entirely to one type; most people represent a combination of types, with one type being more predominant. For example, you can be a pure ectomorph (lean type) or you can be mesomorph (muscular type) with definite tendencies toward the endomorph (bulky) type.

Let's have a closer look at each body type.

Ectomorph

The pure ectomorph is lean and is not at all muscular. Most likely he or she has a fast metabolism and can eat anything without ever getting fat, and for such a type, dieting is not usually a concern.

Mesomorph

The mesomorph has a powerful musculature on a bony framework. Blessed with an ideal metabolism, this type of individual doesn't have to worry about body weight. Also, being naturally active and athletic, the mesomorph can indulge in favorite foods without putting on too much body fat.

Endomorph

This type is characterized by a large bone structure, soft body parts, and a prominent stomach. Having a slow metabolism, the endomorph gains weight easily and has to be very careful with calories, however active he or she is.

Most people who are overweight are unlikely to be pure mesomorph or pure ectomorph. Sometimes an ectomorph will have a rather slow metabolism and will be fat. Most dieters, however, are one of the following types: endomorph, endomorph-mesomorph, or mesomorph-endomorph.

A TYPICAL MEAL

A lot of people who are at their normal weight complain about an oversized stomach. As evidenced by pregnant women, the stomach can be stretched to huge proportions without much gain in fat. For the average person, the stomach can hold about one-and-a-half pounds of food without stretching.

Now let's take a look at a typical American meal.

1 bowl of soup	10 ounces
1 main dish	12 ounces
1 dessert	6 ounces
1 beverage	8 ounces
TOTAL	36 ounces

That's 36 ounces of food—and I'm not taking into consideration the bread and the double servings—compared with 24 ounces the stomach can normally handle. This means that the average eater in America is consuming at least one-third more food than he should—no wonder small, tight, wasp waists are not commonplace anymore. For a serious dieter, the food intake per meal should be ¾ of a pound or 12 ounces, give or take a few ounces depending on your weight, size, and rate of progress.

EATING PREFERENCES: CAVIAR OR PEANUT BUTTER

Eating preferences vary widely around the world. Italians are fond of pasta, Eskimos swear by meat, Chinese eat starchy, oily, high carbohydrate foods (that's supposedly the reason why they wrinkle at a slower rate than we do) and Americans are addicted to fast foods. Meanwhile, primitive tribesmen in the jungles of South America feast on fruits, vegetables, nuts, and roots.

No race in the world can claim a monopoly on health; yet all races have centenarians, which is a tribute to the marvelous adaptive qualities of the human species.

The eating preferences of Americans can be classified into three main categories: vegetarians, health-food fanatics, regular and fast-food eaters.

THE VEGETARIAN

Vegetarianism is the practice of eating only vegetables and plant products for health or moral reasons. There are few true vegetarians around today. Some call themselves ovo-vegetarian, meaning they eat eggs, while others are recognized as lacto-vegetarian, meaning they consume dairy products, but those who eat fish, eggs, and dairy products can't call themselves vegetarians. Surprisingly enough, many so-called vegetarians eat meat once in a while. The problem with vegetarianism is anemia, which is caused by a deficiency of vitamin B-12. Even the late Bernard McFadden (one of the most famous proponents of vegetarianism) once admitted his furtive habit of eating liver more than once in a while. "Liver is a medicine more than a food," he said to justify himself.

I tried vegetarianism for nearly six months but had to give it up because I was feeling too weak to carry on with a demanding training schedule.

Some primitive tribes who appear to be strict vegetarians are really not. They eat bugs, eggs, and even meat occasionally. True vegetarianism is observed in macrobiotic dieting, and deaths have been attributed to such an unbalanced way of eating.

HEALTH-FOOD FANATICS

I must confess that I belonged to the above-mentioned group at one point in my life. It seems to be a normal stage that every health-oriented person goes through at one time or another. Health-food fanatics tend to overlook some facts. Many products sold in a health-food store are not healthy. Some are ineffective, like a placebo, and a few can even be harmful. I know this for a fact because I once worked for one of the biggest natural food companies in the United States.

Take a regular supermarket, for example. Many of the foods they offer are junk but many are good, wholesome, and nutritious. It's the same with a health-food store, although the proportion of junk food found in a health store is considerably less.

Why are junk products found even in a health-food store? Because of the profit motive and a lack of experimentation with some products before they're marketed.

Health-food fanatics (like vegetarians) are a short-lived breed. With time and experience they discover—as I did—the best of both worlds.

REGULAR AND FAST-FOOD EATERS

If you're a regular eater, you're also a fast-food eater. You simply can't ignore fast-foods today. Fast-food places are on every other corner.

The majority of overweight people are in this category of eaters. You don't have to eat out there three times a week to be a fast-food consumer; supermarkets are loaded with fast-foods. Food manufacturers now put pastries on the market that can be eaten right out of the freezer compartment. Is that fast enough for you?

The regular eater doesn't question nutrition patterns; most of the time he or she eats without being hungry, just because the food is there. Not surprisingly, regular eaters believe that they would suffer big headaches if they skipped a meal and that they would die on the spot after a mere three days without food. Moreover, they have a veneration for a slightly-more-than normal amount of fat, which they consider the barometer of their social status depending on whether they got fat on peanut butter sandwiches or caviar and champagne. Indeed, your eating profile can say a lot about you, but how much you can say about it is probably limited to the subjectivity of the matter, as you will see in the next chapters.

10

DR. PEPPER'S LONELY HEARTS CLUB

People are lonely because they build walls instead of bridges. (Joseph F. Newton)

With the publication of a new magazine, a feeble trend has recently begun in the United States (where else?) and it's about the glorification of fat. The message is clear: "Being fat and big is beautiful." The bigger you are the more there is to love (or hate)—a familiar and diplomatic way of giving solace to spouses drowning in fat. There's even a French expression that says literally: "Am I gonna be fatter for this?" which means "Am I gonna be richer for this?"

Despite these suggestions of security in being fat, the fact remains that, for most people, an excess of fat is impractical, unhealthy and ugly.

BEING THIN IS NEVER HAVING TO SAY YOU'RE SORRY

There are many reasons for a fat person to regret his or her obesity. As for the impractical side of being fat, there are all the sports you can't play because you'd be out of breath in less than five minutes. It's also a limiting factor in your social life, not to mention the trouble of shopping for decent clothes. Of course, there are boutiques that carry a line of over-sized garments; unfortunately, they never have exactly what you want or what is really fashionable. Too bad. Buying a car can be another limiting factor—sure you can get into that fancy sports car of your dreams but are you comfortable? And who's going to help you get out of it each time?

Being fat can also be impractical at work. If your work requires you to stand up, your boss might find you sitting down perspiring (to recuperate) once too often for his liking. And although fatness has nothing to do with I.Q., an employer might associate your physical slowness with a mental one. In which case, you could be overlooked for a promotion for someone with more normal physical attributes.

There's also the important aspect of sexual relations. The problem is not so much physical limitations but psychological inhibitions (due to a distorted self-image) interfering with sexual satisfaction.

Additionally, too much fat is unhealthy. The stereotyped image of the happy-go-lucky obese person is a myth. Obesity is associated with high blood pressure, heart disease, arthritis, diabetes, gout, varicose veins, gall bladder, and many other diseases.

Fatness is not only a general impairment but also a burden on blood circulation and its intricate network of veins and capillaries. It is very ugly, as well. Even the corpulent "Baigneuses" of the painter Renoir were praised by only a minority of "upper class" women because at the same time, many of them were strapping themselves in ultra-tight corsets to shape their waistline, hips, and breasts. (To the delight of their male companion, naturally.)

When you're fat you look much older than you are. You're out of proportion and appear awkward and sexually unattractive because the appeals of your sex are hidden in fat. Furthermore, it's very hard to conceal ugly fat when you go out—especially in the summer. And wherever you venture out, there are always kids who make fun of you—behind your pudgy back. Still, you are aware of it and when you can't take anymore of these ego-shattering encounters, you stay home alone. That is truly sad.

LONELINESS AND FATNESS

More and more, urbanization is taking precedence over rural life; the trend is growing so fast that experts predict that by the year 2090 everyone will be living in cities. Yet, despite that strong tendency, people are growing apart and alone. Reports show that in the beginning of the 19th century one in twenty Americans lived alone while today one in five lives alone.

Loneliness is a serious problem and everyone at one time or other has to cope with it. *Living Alone and Liking It* may be a good title for a book but it's easier said than done. The correlation between obesity and loneliness is evident enough. Yet, whether such people are fat because they are lonely or are lonely because they are fat is debatable.

Let's have a look at the eating patterns of a lonely individual.

Lynda's Profile

Name:	Lynda Pepper
Age:	25
Height:	5'1"
Weight:	135 lbs.
Social Status:	Single—lives alone
Work:	Secretary
Pastime:	Reading

The alarm clock goes off. Lynda pushes the snooze button to get an additional ten minutes of sleep. She repeats this process two or three times before she finally gets up. It's too late for breakfast, but she's not usually hungry in the morning anyway. She takes a fast shower, and then starts to dress. In the kitchen she pours herself a tall glass (about 16 ounces) of her favorite cola. Back in her room with the drink, she proceeds to comb her hair and freshen up before rushing to work.

At midmorning break, Lynda has another tall glass of cola and two jelly doughnuts (836 calories, so far).

For lunch (today is payday), Lynda goes to a fast-food pizza place with a friend. For the rest of her work week, she goes out to eat lunch too—alone most of the time.

At midafternoon break, Lynda usually has a glass or two of cola with a bag of potato chips. After work, she picks up some fast-food to eat at home. Unlike many people, she doesn't buy a large grocery once a week; instead, she goes to the supermarket every two or three days to buy food, usually including three king-size bottles of cola.

Lynda's evenings at home are quiet. She doesn't watch much television. She reads a lot, makes a few phone calls, writes a letter once in a while, and eats. She has light meals but she's always nibbling on something, mostly junk food (averaging 3,000–3,500 calories a day).

Lynda has no steady boyfriend and is so lonely that she spends most of her weekends at her parent's house, and each time she visits them she overeats. Her mom is such a good cook!

Most of Lynda's friends are married or going steady. A few years ago she shared an apartment with another girl. Things went okay for a while and then they split up. Lynda still thinks she's too much of an individualist to accept someone else's rules or make concessions of any kind.

She hates being fat and has tried many times to lose weight by participating in sports (jogging, tennis) but without much regularity. She feels it's hard enough being lonely without being on a diet all the time. Yet she's slowly but surely gaining weight and she finds herself going out less and less. She's desperate.

BREAKING THE PATTERN

Lynda must understand that following a diet plan is in fact compatible with her need for individuality. Anyone who's on a diet should be proud of showing determination and willpower.

The first thing Lynda must do is to get up as soon as she wakes up—no more snoozing bouts. After her shower, it would be a good idea for her to go out and walk about a block, breathing deeply. Then if she's hungry, she should have a good breakfast: fruits, oatmeal, cottage cheese, or eggs. If she's not hungry, she can have a small glass (4 to 6 ounces) of unsweetened fruit juice. No more cola drinks.

Mid-morning snack should be a fruit or tomato juice, nothing more. If she still wants to eat out for lunch, she should choose a good restaurant and have a decent low-calorie meal instead of eating fast food.

One of the most important things she must do is grocery shopping once a week only—and no junk food.

She also must stop nibbling during the evening, although a low-calorie snack is permitted.

Her total calories should be in the range of 1,000–1,200, depending on her activities.

She would be wise to reconsider sharing the rent with a girlfriend, but it must be someone who is of normal weight and who has good control of her eating pattern. She also should socialize more than she does, going out at least two or three times a week: learning a foreign language, learning to swim or taking an evening course in something she's interested in. It will do wonders to help her break the loneliness-fatness net in which she's now entangled.

Lynda should realize that her loneliness can be a steady affair (if she so decides) but it's no excuse for being fat and feeling sorry for herself all her life.

11

THE COOKIE MONSTER

Happiness has many roots, but none more important than security. (E. R. Stetlinius, Jr.)

Unemployment, inflation, and divorce are some common causes of insecurity among people today. Underlying all this is the fear of not having food on a regular basis. For the father of a big family who has lost his job, for the young newlywed who just signed a costly mortgage, and for the divorced wife with three kids to support, this feeling of insecurity is a major and understandable concern. Yet some people who don't have such concerns and who are living in average or above-average material comfort are suffering from a deep insecurity about food.

Let's take a look at one of these people.

Orville's Profile

Name:	Orville Cookie
Age:	23
Height:	5'9"
Weight:	210 lbs.
Social Status:	Single, lives with his widowed mother
Work:	Printer
Pastimes:	Eating and watching TV

For four years now Orville has been working as a civil servant in his native city—a secure job for all his working life. Unlike most obese people, Orville appears at first glance as an uncaring, easygoing person. But although he is meticulous in his work and appreciated by his boss, he suffers from insecurity, which is reflected in his eating pattern.

Orville has no social life to speak of but he doesn't care. He likes his life with his mother at home—he even takes his vacations with her, driving her wherever she wants to go—as long as she pays for the food.

At work, Orville usually holds the record for hours of overtime, and he spends more nights at work than at home. His co-workers suspect that money is not the only reason he's such a workaholic. For employees who stay after regular hours, the cafeteria is open and the food is F-R-E-E; and Orville is not only the king of overtime, he's also the undisputed king of overeating. At work his nickname is Cookie Monster. Co-workers often bet on how much pizza Orville will eat at one sitting; since the food is free, he eats anything in sight, as if there were no tomorrow. His diet is a simple one: anything, anywhere, anytime, as long as the food is free or inexpensive. At home there's no problem either. He pays his mother for room and board and eats twice as much as he pays.

Orville doesn't worry about his excess weight but he's not proud of it either; he wouldn't mind being his normal weight if he wouldn't have to cut down his food intake.

BREAKING THE PATTERN

Breaking such a pattern is a big challenge. Of course, he could move out of his mother's house and try living on his own, but this would mean more insecurity and thus more eating. He could indulge in a vigorous sport a couple of times a week, which would increase his self-confidence and burn up some calories. But sports is the last thing on his mind—he's a softy.

Since Orville is not motivated enough to lose his excess weight and his problem has psychological roots, his only road to a lean body may be therapeutic help.

12

THE COMPULSIVE EATER

Necessity has no law. (Benjamin Franklin)

Compulsive preoccupation with food is a tyrannical habit and hard to detect. The compulsive eater can easily fool you into wondering how they got that big because they eat a lot less than their weight suggests and they seem so remote, so detached from mere table pleasures when they eat. Even so, they don't restrict themselves. They have a sample of every food on the table and are usually good conversationalists at mealtimes, as if they wanted to shift your attention from food to other matters. Surprisingly enough, they seem in perfect control of the whole eating process. But all this is a put-on.

The reason a compulsive eater gets so big on so little food is that he eats furtively. He raids the fridge at three in the morning when everyone else is asleep. He has a second breakfast when the kids leave for school. He tells his spouse he's going out to buy the paper and ends up at his favorite hamburger joint.

The compulsive eater goes on binges when he's alone for a good reason. He's so obsessed with food that he feels guilty and thinks everyone around him is conscious of his obsession; so he fakes control over hunger, while in privacy he sins on junk food.

Here's a typical case.

Nancy's Eating Profile

Name:	Nancy Compulsion
Age:	42
Height:	5'5"
Weight:	205 lbs.
Social Status:	Married—three children
Work:	Housewife
Pastimes:	Chatting on the phone, napping, and furtive eating binges.

Nancy is always the first to wake up in the morning. Not that she has to; her husband Paul and her children wouldn't mind preparing their own breakfast. Setting up breakfast for her family is like going to church on Sunday—a must, a duty. For her first meal of the day, Nancy is never hungry; that's what she tells her family; nevertheless, she always has a little something with them. At eight o'clock when everybody's gone, she usually goes back to sleep for an hour or so. When she gets up she has an incredible breakfast that puts more than muscle on her.

After her first tremendous eating bout of the day, Nancy usually watches Joe Smiley's morning show on the tube. Then she gets dressed and does some chores or calls a friend. At eleven-thirty she starts cooking lunch while nibbling on every food she puts her hands on. When her family comes home, she serves them generously and takes a small portion for herself. She always has a small-to-medium serving of dessert, pretending to her children that it's no use for her to diet because she has a hormonal malfunction or something to that effect. But when everyone's back at school and work, the remains of the Swiss chocolate cake disappear magically and some of that vanilla ice cream in the freezer compartment seems to melt away. Time for another nap—a natural thing to do after a hearty meal.

When Nancy wakes up around one-thirty, she goes downtown to do some shopping or visit a friend. In either case she has a high calorie snack—not a large amount of food, just enough concentrated calories to keep her going until dinner. Dinner at home is another cover-up for her compulsive eating pattern. But eating after dinner is more tricky because her husband and children are home. Nevertheless, by frequent trips to the kitchen and without ever sitting down to eat, she manages to cram many hundreds of calories. Then when the children are asleep, she snacks on cheese and crackers with her husband while watching the news.

As you can see, that's a lot of calories for someone who has a slow metabolism and doesn't work. (Nancy also wakes up at night to go to the bathroom and has a clumsy way of stumbling upon the fridge each time around.)

BREAKING THE PATTERN

Such a typical pattern of compulsive eating is hard to break, but it can be done and doesn't necessarily require the help of a therapist. Nancy is definitely unhappy with her life; she has very little self-esteem and feels guilty after each eating binge. It seems to her that her whole life revolves around overeating in secrecy, chatting on the phone, and napping. She should consider getting a job, doing exercises, or going to yoga classes to build up her self-image. She must go on a diet that would permit her to indulge in her favorite food at times and allow enough protein to ward off her craving for sweets—the Cheater's Diet fills those needs perfectly, as you will see later. Moreover, it would be a good idea for her to get involved in a non-profit social organization to take her mind off food for a while. Finally, reading books on mind control, self-hypnosis, and behavioral therapy would definitely help in breaking this eating pattern forever.

13

THE LAZY DIETER

It is hard to fail but it is worse to never have tried to succeed. In this life we get nothing save by effort. (Theodore Roosevelt)

When you succeed in anything that is worthwhile in life, there's always a lot of people around you who want to know how you did it. Unfortunately no one surrounds the loser to ask him how come he blew it. That's why many unsuccessful would-be dieters give you the usual litany of excuses before you even ask them anything, such as:

"My father was a big man"; "I've got a glandular problem"; "I don't have time"; "I don't eat much"; "It's the water in my tissues"; "I can't follow a diet while my wife is eating all she wants"; "I'm a cook, I can't diet"; "I work on night shift so it's hard to diet for very long."

All these individuals have three things in common:

1. They don't really want to get rid of their extra fat.
2. They think it will take sacrifices and hard work to do so.
3. They are too lazy to get the task done.

Lazy dieters are legion in number; their favorite statement begins with: "I would like to lose weight but . . . "

Let's take a close look at a lazy dieter.

Jim's Profile

Name:	Jim Lazy
Age:	27
Height:	5'10"
Weight:	220 lbs.
Social Status:	Newlywed
Work:	School Teacher
Pastimes:	Drinking beer and fishing

Lazy-bones Jim they used to call him at school. Even then, he showed all the characteristics of the perfect endomorph. He would spend his recreation time sitting in a corner with some other sluggish schoolmates munching on peanuts and potato chips. But although he was lazy, he was no dummy. He finished school with high marks and easily earned a teaching degree in mathematics. Since he was good with numbers, Jim had no problem figuring out that teaching would leave him two full months with nothing to do—nothing except fishing and drinking beer.

After a few years of this sedentary life, Jim's weight rose to a whopping 245 pounds. Then one day he was rushed to the hospital for an appendectomy. A month after his surgery, Jim's weight had stablized around 220. During his short stay at the hospital, he had lost ten pounds and the scare of the operation gave him enough willpower to cut down on foods until he shed another fifteen pounds. But at 220 he is still 30 to 40 pounds over his normal weight.

Jim never has breakfast if his wife isn't up to prepare it. He drives to work even though school is only five blocks from his home. At mid-morning he usually snacks on two or three doughnuts and a cup of coffee. At lunch time he drives home where his wife has cooked a typical high-calorie meal. Later in the afternoon, he snacks on a few pops and a bag of potato chips, and his dinner is another high-calorie meal.

In the evening, Jim generally drives to his favorite tavern (a five-minute walk) to meet his buddies. They usually close the place. Back home, Jim eats a pizza or Chinese food while watching the late movie. And the next morning, the cycle begins again.

Dieting is definitely not Jim's forte. Nevertheless, he is a proud man and would like to reduce his weight, but he is still looking for the easiest way. One day his wife remarks that he looks pregnant. That does it.

His neighbor Kevin works out with weights, and he has often invited Jim to train with him. So Jim starts to train in earnest—for a while. A very short while. He starts missing training sessions under the pretext of having a sprained ankle or feeling sick. But he's feeling well enough to make it to the tavern and exercise his elbow. So much for laziness.

BREAKING THE PATTERN

First, forgetting the tavern is a must, there's no need for therapy. All Jim has to do is build up enough energy to shake off his laziness. He should stick around with his friend Kevin more often. Exercise is indeed the best cure for laziness—the more you do the more you want to do. He also should leave his car home and walk to work. And his late evening eating habits must end so that he will be hungry enough to eat a decent breakfast and pass up the mid-morning coffee and doughnuts.

Fortunately for Jim, the Cheater's Diet has been conceived with lazy, weak-willed food lovers in mind.

14

THE IGNORANT DIETER

All wish to possess knowledge, but few, comparatively speaking, are willing to pay the price. (Juvenal)

Fifty percent of all unsuccessful dieters are ignorant about dieting. How can this be? With all the information available today, no one should be ignorant about a subject that matters to them. The problem with many dieters is that they follow any cheap diet they find in a comic book. But those cheap diets—and most of the not-so-cheap ones—generally provide only a regular menu and tell when and when you should not follow it. Such diets perpetuate the most common myths about foods so as not to scare away any potential dieter.

Nowhere in those booklets will you find information about basic metabolism, digestion, health in general, and the need for exercise. Nor will they explore or discuss any controversial subject related to dieting, and all this for a good reason: not because they think that dieters are pea-brained individuals who wouldn't understand what it's all about but because they themselves have no pertinent experience beyond having lost a few pounds once. Even if a person has lost 100 pounds of fat in only three months, that's no sure-fire indication that he or she knows a lot about the art of dieting and related topics. It may well be that he simply ate considerably less and burned more energy during a certain period of time.

Another reason for dietetic ignorance is lack of academic interest in nutrition. As a result, the average person comes out of school knowing more about the mechanics and care of a car than the mechanics and nutritional processes of his own body. And after leaving school, how many people—on their own—study nutrition, biology, and other topics related to the human body. Unfortunately, the human machine doesn't come with an owner's manual.

The pattern of the ignorant dieter is not complicated. He uses the buck-shot technique, mixing together the most popular myths and, when in doubt, he relies on his judgment.

The Ignorant Dieter

Let's meet an average ignorant dieter.

Diane's Profile

Name:	Diane Ignorant
Age:	29
Height:	5'8"
Weight:	205 lbs.
Social Status:	Married—Two children
Work:	Bank employee
Pastimes:	TV and camping

Not until Diane ballooned to 180 pounds did she learn that potatoes are not a concentrated source of calories but the margarine that she puts liberally on her vegetables is. Her shock was even greater when she reached 185 and found that the grapefruit juice she was drinking did nothing to burn all the fats she was eating; instead, it added calories to her diet. At 190 pounds Diane discovered that her weekly aerobic dance classes were more than neutralized by the two or three pops she was drinking to replace her lost fluid; all that time she thought that pop was only water and a bit of sugar. Then she went on four quarts of water a day to lose weight by elimination. Her mother had learned about the diet from TV and had phoned to tell her about it. After a month on this diet and endless trips to the bathroom, she still weighed 195 pounds. She was desperate. Her mother finally persuaded her to forget about diets altogether because a doctor had brought out a new theory: Obese people are born that way and nothing can be done to reverse their momentum toward gaining weight.

The theory does make sense, reasoned Diane; after all, her grandmother was obese and had eaten like a bird (a vulture probably) most of her life. So, resigned, Diane started eating liberally again and soon reached 205 pounds. Then one summer morning, while on a camping vacation with her husband and kids, she woke up to go to the john. After a short spurt of urine, she felt a burning sensation in her lower back and almost fainted. Her husband rushed her to the hospital, where her suffering was diagnosed as kidney stones. A few weeks after the operation, her doctor investigated her eating habits. He was bewildered when she candidly mentioned eating a king-size jar of mayonnaise each weekend all by herself. The doctor said that this habit of hers coupled with her smoking a pack of cigarettes a day might have a lot to do with the presence of stones in her body. So Diane started smoking low-tar cigarettes and replaced mayonnaise with margarine.

BREAKING THE PATTERN

The first step in the right direction for Diane would be to stop listening to people around her. She also would do well to attend conferences on nutrition and start reading serious books on biology and dieting. In short, she must change her old-wives'-tales approach to dieting to a more scientific, up-to-date one if she really wants to get back to her normal weight. For in the case of an ignorant dieter, it's not simply breaking an eating pattern but developing a *learning* pattern.

15

THE ON-AND-OFF DIETER

Everything comes to him who hustles while he waits. (Thomas A. Edison)

The On-and-Off Dieter is afflicted by what I call the *yo-yo syndrome*. Unlike the ignorant dieter he knows the basics of nutrition in relation to dieting, and when he sets his mind on losing weight he succeeds most of the time, only to put it back on as fast as he has lost it. He has the knowledge but lacks consistency. The usual regular-straight diet bores him to death. What he needs is variety and a frequent change of pace.

Usually the dieting sprees of such individuals follow a definite cycle that may be related to the seasons. This cycle may also be influenced by strong emotional disturbances. Although this dieter is successful at times, his dieting cycle never lasts long enough for him to reach his desired weight. Yet he's an optimist and always thinks that the next time around he will finally reach his goal.

James's Profile

Name:	James Onandoff
Age:	31
Height:	6'1"
Weight:	245 lbs.
Social Status:	Divorced
Work:	Police officer
Pastimes:	Jogging and swimming

Each spring James is afflicted by jogger's fever, and the cure is always the same: He goes to a sports store and buys a pair of running shoes and a sweat suit. It might be a psychological thing with him, but over the years he felt that he had to start the running season with a new outfit. (He never runs indoors.) So beginning in April, James starts jogging every day until he builds up his capacity to run from two to five miles, depending on his energy level. He also cuts his beer intake down to almost nothing and shops in a health-food store for vitamin E, wheat germ oil, granola cereals, and other health goodies. At this point, James knows he's on his way to shedding the winter spread he has accumulated. At 245 pounds he is 30 pounds over his best body weight of 215, which he usually reaches by July.

Then something mysterious happens. The weather seems too hot to run, beer finds its way to his stomach more often, and thoughts of the coming summer vacation drain his will to train and diet.

When James' vacation is over he is up to around 230 lbs. He tries—unsuccessfully—to resume his jogging and dieting. Deep inside James knows the reason for his failure. It's not the exercise part that he dreads most but the diet that goes with it. He can't diet for long without getting bored; he can't stay away from a double cheese lasagna at least once a week.

Yet when September comes, it's time for jogging and dieting again because his weight is up to his initial 245 lbs. This bout of enthusiasm will last until December. Then he's trapped in the Christmas blues and loses all interest in dieting. By mid-January he will go to the local pool about twice a week but he's not motivated enough to diet again. So when spring comes, James still weighs 245 or a bit more and the cycle starts all over again, never permitting him to reach his ideal weight and keep it under control.

BREAKING THE PATTERN

James' problem is in his too-much-too-soon approach. He should run only every other day and make it a year-round habit. That doesn't mean he can't take a break for two weeks or so, but if he does he *must* set the exact date at which he will resume his diet and exercise program and unconditionally stick to it. Moreover, James shouldn't let his feelings and emotions get in the way. Dieting and exercise are things he hates to do and yet he hates himself for not doing them. He should schedule a less stringent diet for himself and a more regular exercise program and forget his emotional dilemma.

Basically a good diet never changes: It's relatively low in calories and provides a variety of fresh, natural foods. Success is sweet but lasting success is even sweeter.

Part III

The Solution

16

FASTING TO LOSE WEIGHT

Complete abstinence is easier than perfect moderation. (St. Augustine)

Fasting has been around for a long time. It often has a religious basis, but has also been used as a means of protest by political prisoners and protestors. A long time ago, cavemen were forced to fast for days because of the harsh conditions of their life. Jesus himself went to the desert and fasted for 40 days. Mahatma Gandhi, the late spiritual leader of India, fasted more than once. There is also a legend about a Roman emperor who, concluding that the best time to die was when one has reached happiness, fasted until he died. Several years ago in an Ireland prison, Bobby Sands and his companions died from fasting. Such examples of long fasts had nothing to do with losing weight; they were of a spiritual or ideological nature.

WHAT IS FASTING?

Fasting means abstaining from food. In its general definition, food means anything that nourishes the body and contributes to the maintenance of life, such as proteins, fats and carbohydrates, all of which contain calories. Many people have the impression they are fasting when the only thing they are doing is restraining their food intake. You can say you have fasted when the only thing you swallowed for at least 24 hours was water. Anything else is not a fast. Even if you only chew gum, you're not fasting. Gum contains calories.

I remember when one of my friends who was on the fat side proudly announced that he had fasted for seven days in a row. In disbelief I started asking him questions and found out that he had eaten fruits for breakfast, vegetable juice for lunch, and soup for supper. Anyone could live for years eating that way. Some vegetarians do just that. You can't call that fasting. It's just a different, limited way of eating.

The main reason fasting is not a good way to lose body weight is because it puts a stress on the body and mind. (Most people are so condi-

Fasting to Lose Weight

tioned to eating three big meals a day that they think if they go three days without food they'll die.) Also, fasting is impractical. You can't fast for long if you work. After only one day without food you'll start feeling chilly, dizzy, and obsessed about food. Furthermore your family and friends will start putting incredible pressure on you to resume eating because they care for you. All this makes fasting extremely difficult for anyone who tries it—unless he lives in a monastery.

Suppose you weigh yourself after one day of fasting and the scale shows a three-pound loss. You may be misled into thinking that you've lost three pounds of fat but that isn't so. The body can hold a lot more food (fluids and solids) than you think. Weight reduction will have been mostly caused by dehydration and an empty stomach. In fact, you'll have lost only a few ounces of real fat. So if you have a lot of pounds to lose, many weeks are required to do the task. But you still have to earn a living, don't you? Oh, sure, during your vacation you could fast under a doctor's supervision but even then fasting could be detrimental. The bottom line is, the fatter you are, the more dangerous a long fast can be. Let's face it, if you are obese you must be into junk food. There's no way around it. No one gets fat eating vegetables, fruits, and lean meat. So if you are undernourished—but overfed with empty calories, thus fat—and you start fasting suddenly, you will further deprive your body. You will be playing Russian roulette.

I knew an obese man who went to a health resort to reduce his weight through a long fast. He succeeded. He also died in the process 38 days later. Putting it mildly, a long fast is like an electroshock in medicine. It's the last recourse.

THE BEST WAY TO FAST

Does this mean fasting has no value at all?

Quite the contrary. The best thing you can do when you have reached your normal body weight is to fast one day each week—not to make sure you don't gain back weight, but to give your overworked internal organs a beneficial rest. Laboratory experiments with rats have shown that fasting one day a week causes a substantial increase in their longevity. Do you think free animals in the woods eat regularly seven days out of seven? Of course not! Still, in proportion to our life expectancy, they live twice as long as we do.

A short fast—from one to no more than three days—is the best way to rest and clean your whole system. But one day fasts are more practical; you don't have to stop working to do it. For a two- or three-day fast, I would recommend that you retire to a quiet place, such as a beach house or a cabin in the woods. You can do that alone or with a friend who also wants to fast. The aim is to relax and keep your mind off foods by creating a diversion. You can play cards, chess, or just converse. Be sure to drink a lot of fresh water, even if you aren't thirsty, to prevent dehydration and provide better elimination of body toxins.

Let's go through a preview of a typical one-day fast.

You wake up early in the morning. You're not that hungry. You skip breakfast—no big deal. And you rush (sorry, stroll) to work.

At the mid-morning coffee break, you sip a tall glass of cool water—and continue sipping even though your co-workers give you funny looks. Lunch time: You don't show up at the cafeteria as usual; you go for a walk instead. A close friend follows you to inquire if you're sick. No, you assure him, you're only fasting for a day.

In the late afternoon you start feeling chilly, so you borrow a wool sweater from someone. The entire office staff knows by now that you're on a fast. You must be a weirdo to harm your body like this, they think. Nevertheless, you carry on with determination until five o'clock and finally make it home. Now you think you're safe. But this is the day your wife cooks your favorite dish—she's forgotten that you are fasting. You drink another tall glass of water and end up in the living room reading the newspaper while your wife and kids sit down for a terrific meal. That's the tough part. That's where you can fail. Fortunately you just got a great idea to ward off temptation. You go to the movies. Nine-thirty you're back. The children are asleep and you sit down in front of the tube with your wife. You think you have it made. But your wife goes to the kitchen and comes back with an appetizing double-decker sandwich—a favorite of yours. Heroically, you kiss your wife goodnight, reach for another tall glass of water to stop that rumbling in your stomach, and go to bed. But you can't sleep. Your stomach is crying for food. Finally, an hour later, you fall into a light sleep. At five in the morning you're sitting up in bed, your eyeballs hanging from their sockets. You stumble out of bed and finally steady yourself. Never in your life have you felt so light on your feet. You are feeling proud to have made it—one day without any food, just tap water.

Still interested in fasting? And that's for only one day. Okay, I will concede it's not a cinch. But let's look at the immediate rewards of a one-day fast. If you resume eating intelligently the day after a fast, the first thing you will notice is an increase in energy. The next forty-eight hours will find you bursting with pep. Besides, your whole perception of life will be more acute. Your senses—vision, smell, taste, and touch—will be more intense than ever. If a big meal puts you to sleep like a drug, fasting, on the other hand, will heighten your senses dramatically. You should experience this feeling at least once in your life. The longest I've ever fasted was three-and-a-half days. I experienced no side effects whatsoever. I felt just great and very much alive. I will probably do it again, at the right time and in the right place.

As I write this, it's Sunday afternoon. I've skipped breakfast and lunch, as I do most Sundays. Around dinner time I'll go for a walk or bike ride. Tonight, if I can't bear the pressure anymore, I'll go to the movies to keep my mind off food.

When you are in shape and you eat well, and have reached your normal body weight, and you're mentally ready for it, a short fast is one of the healthiest practices you can indulge in. It will boost your battery (nervous system) like nothing else can. But remember that a long fast is not a good solution for losing weight in an easy, and most of all, healthy way.

17

THE FRENCH CONNECTION

Some remedies are worse than the diseases. (Publilius Syrus)

Another hazardous way of losing weight is what I call the French Connection, or the use of drugs, if you like. Generally speaking, a drug is a substance used as a medicine to treat disease. And it can be either addictive or not. Some people are truly illogical—it's incredible. They are fanatical about putting only the manufacturer's recommended oil into their car. Yet these same people—who have never gulped down anything stronger than jalepeño peppers—think nothing of ingesting drugs strong enough to kill a gorilla. All this for the sake of losing only a few extra pounds of fat sometimes. Just because a crackpot in a laboratory has found a miracle drug that burns fat (naturally he hasn't tried it himself, *you are the guinea pig*) doesn't mean you have to rush to your doctor's office for a prescription. Think twice before swallowing any drug; your health is at stake, not the physician's.

JANET THE SPEED FREAK

One winter morning, Janet rolled her 160 pounds out of bed. She was depressed. Her husband had called the night before telling her he wouldn't come home to sleep because he had to work overtime on the night shift. But the reflection of her overloaded five-foot-three-frame in the mirror convinced her that her husband's excuse was a fishy one, especially for a Friday night.

The following week Janet ended up in her doctor's office. She told him she had to lose weight fast, and the doctor tried to talk her into dieting. Janet started crying and explained to him that she had to lose weight in a hurry because her marriage was on the rocks and surely those little pink pills would do the trick. Touched, the physician prescribed a one-month supply of amphetamines that she could renew only once. Janet took the pills diligently for two months and eureka! She was down to 128 pounds. She was delighted and so was her husband who shunned overtime for a while. Of course she was still plump and her skin was loose around the waist, but with a few more weeks on the pills and some exercise, everything would be okay.

Janet went back to her doctor to get another prescription. He refused, explaining that amphetamines shouldn't be taken regularly because they could be detrimental to the heart and nervous system. Instead he gave her a copy of a classical, boring-to-death diet. Halfheartedly Janet tried the doctor's diet. About two weeks later, she was back to 135 pounds, a gain of eight pounds. Now panic got the best of her. She was afraid her husband might start working overtime again. Then she remembered her sister was going out with a weird guy who was supposed to be in real estate. She also remembered him hinting that he could deliver just about any kind of "goods." So Janet got in touch with her sister's boyfriend and a few days later she had a jar full of amphetamines. She upped the dosage to two a day instead of one as prescribed by the doctor; she had some catching up to do, she thought.

One month of this regimen brought Janet's weight to a slim 105 pounds—a loss of 30 pounds. She was satisfied with that body weight, but she didn't want to gain back any ugly fat. So she kept taking one pill a day to cut her appetite down. But she felt grouchy and the loose skin around her waist was nothing to be proud of. Also, her red-popped eyes and the brown bags underneath them made her look ready for the vultures. Janet went into a deep depression. Finally her husband left her.

Not a happy ending yet a true one. Taking amphetamines or "speed" of any kind, however small the amount, is definitely not a wise solution for losing weight.

DIURETICS

Another phony approach to losing weight is diuretic drugs. They will only make you pee like a heavy beer drinker and overwork your kidneys. If you take an excess of calories, diuretics or not, you will stay fat. *You can't pee the calories away.* It just doesn't work that way.

INJECTIONS

Not too long ago, two lovely women of my acquaintance decided to open a gym that would cater to women only. Since they were lacking in experience on how to run a gym, they asked if I would help them start their new business. I agreed to spare an afternoon for their project. As they were showing me around the gym, which wasn't officially open yet, we entered a small room furnished only with a desk and chair. They told me this was the doctor's office and it was already in operation. Twice a week the doc showed up and gave women (willing to pay twenty dollars a shot) injections of "natural" enzymes into their thighs. Now this process was supposed to "eat" the cellulite away. Surely, everyone knows that enzymes are the meanest eaters in the world. You may have seen a laundry ad on TV that shows enzymes eating dirt faster than piranhas eat flesh. Isn't it comforting to know that those little buggers can do the same for your thighs, ladies?

One look at the garbage pail beside the doctor's desk assured me that he had been very busy lately. However, with any injection your body receives, the risk is twofold: first, there's a risk of infection due to the syringe itself, and second, there's a risk of a rejection or an allergic reaction due to an unfamiliar element in your body.

In case you have a lot of money to throw away or you are a health "junkie," let me add one more thing. Injections don't work at all. I saw a woman who had been on the treatment for nearly six months and she was the first to admit she had wasted a lot of money for nothing. Besides, most substances you inject into your body (including the popular vitamin B-12) are detrimental to some degree. An injection is unnatural for your body. It's a poison.

The next case of weight reduction I want to talk about is the laziest and fastest way to remove fat from your stomach. All you need to accomplish this feat is an anesthetist, a surgeon, a scalpel, and a gallstones diagnosis. After the surgeon has removed your gallbladder, he takes his magic scalpel and cleans your stomach of all superfluous fat. Wonderful. Perhaps you won't believe this but some obese people are actually looking for ways to end up on the operating table to get rid of their fat. And the general anesthesia is done with a powerful drug.

Each time you enter an operating room you are taking some risks. There's always the possibility of internal complications and hospital staffs are only human.

The most extreme case of weight reduction I've heard of has nothing to do with drugs but is nevertheless an artificial, radical, and drastic measure. A big, fat guy, unable to lose weight (the Cheater's Diet wasn't out yet) decided to get his jaws wired closed, leaving only a small hole between his teeth so he could drink with a straw. Fortunately, it worked.

In case you're not interested in having your jaws wired or parts of your stomach removed, just turn to the next chapter for a sane solution: the Cheater's Diet.

18

THE CHEATER'S DIET

The pleasures of the palate deal with us like the Egyptian thieves, who strangle those whom they embrace. (Seneca)

This is it—The Cheater's Diet! Although I have been very impatient to write this chapter—the most important one in the book—I've let the ideas build up slowly to give this chapter its fullest meaning.

The Cheater's Diet's only drawback may be that it will look too simple to be effective for some people. But for those who think that life shouldn't be complicated, take heed: the revolutionary Cheater's Diet is here to last. Its secret resides in three words: *cheaper, easier, faster*. And the results are permanent. When you finish with this book, you'll be on a healthy, effective diet for the rest of your life.

The Cheater's Diet is cheaper than other diets because you have nothing extra to buy. No gadget, apparatus, liquid, scale, utensil, or complimentary book. It's also cheaper because it requires no special or expensive food—just regular foods prepared in a *new* way. Moreover, the Cheater's Diet is a medium protein diet. And because proteins are quite expensive, it's cheaper than high protein diets that require you to eat three servings of meat daily.

As will be explained in Chapter 29, food supplements are optional. They do not play a major role in this diet. You can lose all the weight you want and stay that way without ever knowing what a supplement looks like. Supplements should be looked on as a luxury for health-minded individuals, like an extra insurance premium. Food supplements will not speed up the losing process per se, although they make regular dieting easier between cheating meals. If you decided on investing some money on supplements as part of your Cheater's Diet program, you will save in the long run. You will significantly reduce your medical bill and have more energy at work. And you will save on the amount of food for your cheating meals because of better long-term nutrition.

Anyone from 7 to 77 can follow the Cheater's Diet. You don't have to be strong willed to get results with it. Because cheating is *a must* in order to lose weight, this diet is literally a piece of cake. In fact, it's so easy that once you get accustomed to it, you'll stick to it for the rest of your life.

The Cheater's Diet also lets you lose weight at your own rate. The regularly scheduled cheating meals make it easier for you to eat less between binges. And your enthusiasm for the diet will always be at a peak.

In the weight-losing game, three questions are most often asked by new dieters:

1. How do I do it?
2. How long will it take before I reach my ideal weight?
3. What happens if I stop dieting?

The Cheater's Diet doesn't guarantee that you'll lose so many pounds in so many days. *No diet can do that.* There are too many imponderables involved. Human beings are not machines. Dieting is an art form, the results having to do with human effort, aesthetic value, and a high conception of beauty. All successful dieters can rightfully call themselves artists, for they are the sculptors of their own body. Their tools are food, exercise, and willpower. Artists are proud of their portrayals of the human form. Why then shouldn't you be proud of transforming your body into a work of art, or at least into a more aesthetic form?

The only guarantee the Cheater's Diet can give you is that if you follow it the chances of losing all the fat you want are excellent. Why? Only about one obese person in a hundred can't lose weight because of hormonal problems. And there are a lot more people wanting to lose a mere five or ten pounds of unwanted fat than there are obese people. So mathematically speaking, your chances of reducing are excellent.

HOW, WHEN, WHY

One morning a few years ago, I got on the scale and found out I weighed 188 pounds. Being 5'8" and the mesomorph-ectomorph type, I wasn't pudgy, chubby, or corpulent. I was simply overweight and I wasn't afraid to acknowledge it. The extra fat was the result of having bulked up to compete in wristwrestling as a middleweight contender. Then one day I received an invitation to compete in the World Wristwrestling Championship in Kansas City. I decided to compete but not in the middleweight class, since I wasn't a natural middleweight. Instead, I decided to enter the lightweight class—under 160 pounds. I had five weeks before the contest to lose some 30 pounds. I thought I could do it if I found an easy way to diet for those five weeks while keeping my energy up for two-hour training sessions, four times a week. I must state at this point that although I didn't smoke or drink, I loved to eat. And I wasn't about to eat tuna fish until it came out of my pores or eat salad until my eyes turned green.

So I sat down and in a couple of days devised a new diet. I had no name for it then. It was just "my" diet and I hoped it would work. I made it a low-fat diet to cut down on unnecessary calories, and medium carbohydrates to have enough energy and ensure a better protein utilization as well as medium protein to ensure a normal blood sugar level to ward off the depressed feeling common to most dieters on a low-protein diet.

I wanted this new diet of mine to be healthy; no junk foods. That's what I thought at first. Then the idea of introducing a cheating meal dawned on me. An occasional cheating meal wouldn't negate the effect of my regular diet and would do a lot of good for keeping my spirits high. Besides, such a meal would be high in carbohydrates and would give me added energy for the next few days.

So, when my decision to add cheating meals to my diet was taken, the only thing I had to do was figure out how many days of straight eating I should leave between the binges. Taking into account my medium metabolism and the deadline I had to respect to reach my goal, I came up with one cheating meal every four days. I knew this tactic would ensure a substantial weight loss without impairing my energy level or affecting my mood. I was elated. Everything worked out as I had planned. Less than five weeks later, in Kansas City, I weighed in at 158 pounds—a total loss of 30 pounds. Unfortunately, I didn't win in my weight class, but at least the Cheater's Diet was born.

TESTING MY PHILOSOPHY

Back to work at my gym, I decided that further testing of my newfound diet would be a good idea, since I wanted to be sure of the effectiveness and practicality of my diet. I kept things more or less secret. I chose to have women only for this experimental project (as a group they have more willpower and show more seriousness about dieting than men). I also made a point of selecting women who were having a hard time losing weight with my old approach of eat-less-of-everything-and-exercise-will-do-the-rest. I explained to them individually the basic theory behind the Cheater's Diet and asked them to keep the experiment a secret for the two months it would last, and they would report to me every week on how they were doing. Together we made slight modifications along the way.

At the two-month deadline, all of them had lost more weight than in the previous two-month session and then were delighted with the results—not so much because they had lost a few more pounds than they would have with the old way but mainly because it had been *so easy*. They reported not having the impression of being on a real diet, and their attitude was more positive. In short, they felt that the Cheater's Diet was exciting, simple, and more effective than any other diet they had ever been on. These results were conclusive enough for me. The Cheater's Diet was brought to the other gym members with the same positive results.

HOW IT WORKS

Basically the Cheater's Diet is a healthy low-calorie diet with a not-so-healthy cheating meal every four days. I say a not-so-healthy meal because most people prefer to cheat on junk food. But you can also cheat on healthier high calorie food like cream, peanut butter, butter, and cheese. Most of my cheating meals are made up of such food. Once in a while I will cheat on pizza, hamburgers, French fries, or ice cream. However, there are a few junk foods I will rarely or never eat; they include colas, hot dogs, coffee, tea, margarine, and synthetic orange juice.

Any junk food eaten once or twice a week won't hurt you; it's what you put into your body on a *daily* basis that can make or break you. For example, suppose there are two identical seven-year-old twins and one of them ate a candy bar every day while the other ate seven candy bars once a week. Everything else being equal, which one do you think would end up with more cavities? It's the same with food. Eating junk food once in a while has no effect on your health; because of the irregularity factor they don't add up.

Now let's talk about the mathematics of calories. To make things easier to understand, we'll estimate how much you could lose on a ten-day cycle with the Cheater's Diet.

Suppose you are now eating about 2,200 calories a day and this amount is keeping your weight stable. During a ten-day period you'd eat 22,000 calories.

(10 days × 2,200 calories = 22,000 calories)

With the Cheater's Diet you'd eat around 1,000 calories a day for a total of 10,000 over a ten-day period.

(10 days × 1,000 calories = 10,000 calories)

Thus, on a ten-day cycle you will save 12,000 calories.

(22,000 calories − 10,000 calories = 12,000 calories)

So, from the 12,000 calories you save on your ten-day cycle, you subtract 1,500 extra calories for the two cheating meals and you will save 10,500 calories.

(12,000 calories − 1,500 = 10,500 calories)

These 10,500 calories you saved would amount to a 3-lb. loss in body fat (one pound of fat being equal to 3,500 calories).

(10,500 calories ÷ 3,500 = 3 pounds lost)

On a ten-day cycle you are allowed two cheating meals, which would roughly amount to 1,500 calories over your regular meal allotment (that's about 350 calories a meal if you ate three meals a day). So two regular meals of 350 calories total 700 calories. Add to this figure 1,500 calories for cheating and you get 2,200 calories for your two cheating meals or 1,100 for each cheating meal, which is plenty for most dieters. And, if you exercised half an hour a day or one hour every other day, you would lose an additional pound at the end of the ten-day cycle.

So if you add the three pounds lost with the Cheater's Diet to the one pound lost from exercising, you have a four-lb. loss of body fat every ten days, or 12 pounds a month—or 36 pounds for three months. That's a lot of fat to lose. (Try to imagine 36 pounds of butter piled up on your kitchen table!)

Don't be frightened by those figures; they are only a guide to show how the diet works. You won't have to count calories on a daily basis and with exact precision. When you start with the Cheater's Diet you try to eat about 1,000 calories a day. It could be 900 or 1,200. You don't have to be a fanatic about it. Then after the first ten-day cycle, you will be able to evaluate the rate at which you are losing weight; the only thing you have to do is eat a bit more or less, depending on how your weight goes.

Later in this chapter you'll find a detailed sample of a regular eating day that averages 1,000 calories.

FOOD GROUPS

Meat Group

The Cheater's Diet is a medium protein diet. You need vitamin B-12 from animal protein if you want to be strong and healthy. Meat and fish are the best sources of this vitamin. Dairy products contain some and vegetables have only traces. Ever wonder why the grass grows so fast after it rains? Rain water contains vitamin B-12.

The Cheater's Diet allows all kinds of lean meats: chicken, veal, turkey, lamb, etc. As a rule, beef is not permitted because it contains about twice as many calories as an equal portion of chicken. Giblets are out too because they are loaded with fat. So is pork, bacon, ham, and sausages.

The meat must be cooked without butter or oil. Meat broiled with fresh vegetables is okay. Meat simmered in water with seasonings makes a nice boullion.

Lean fish is permitted (sole, snapper, etc.), and so is tuna packed in water. Lobster and shrimp are allowed when eaten with natural seasonings, such as lime, instead of the regular sauces sold in supermarkets.

Nuts can be eaten but they must be fresh and plain—unsalted, unroasted, and unprocessed in any way; but, eat them sparingly.

Eggs are on the regular menu of the Cheater's Diet. They can be soft or hard boiled, poached or made into a delicious omelette. (No milk in your omelette; cold water will do just fine.)

If in doubt as to the caloric content of some meat or fish, check the calorie chart in this book.

Vegetables—Fruit Group

All vegetables are allowed in your new diet, provided they are fresh. They can be eaten raw or cooked. Steam-cooked is best but water-cooked is acceptable. Frozen vegetables contain a lot of sodium; try to avoid them as a rule. Canned vegetables also contain a lot of sodium and sometimes, white sugar. So your best bet is to stick to fresh unprocessed vegetables.

All fresh fruits are permitted, except avocado (too high in calories). All dried fruits are forbidden. So are most canned and frozen fruits, except for the few that are unsweetened and packed in their own natural juices.

Bread—Cereal Group

Sorry folks but pasta is a big no-no in the Cheater's Diet—save pasta for your cheating meals.

The best cereals are oatmeal, cornmeal, wheatgerm, shredded wheat (100 percent), and cream of wheat. These cereals should be untoasted and unsweetened. Add the flavoring yourself: sliced fresh fruits, a dash of cinnamon, and a teaspoonful of honey. Regular sugar-loaded children's cereals have no place in your regular meals. Avoid the cornflakes variety; even unsweetened, they are way too high in sodium.

Pancakes, including those with wholesome ingredients, are forbidden for the same reason as pasta. Those two dishes are plain, dry, and tasteless without gravy or syrup; the temptation would be too strong. So eat pancakes and pasta with everything you want on them but only on a scheduled cheating meal.

As for bread, stick with 100 percent whole wheat, rye, or any kind of whole grain bread.

Milk—Cheese Group

Dairy products are an important part of any diet. A major source of calcium, they also provide vitamins A, B6, B12, and usually vitamin D. Still, this food group is probably the most controversial of the four basic food groups. For one thing, most people in the world don't consume milk products on a regular daily basis as we Americans do. Moreover, milk is often considered "the" food for babies. Also most milk products are high in fat (butter is about 80 percent fat while cream rates between 10 to 35 percent) and they lack fiber.

This doesn't mean that all dairy products should be regarded as poison. Some dairy products, such as the following, are needed in the regular part of the Cheater's Diet to add welcome variety and ensure better nutrition:

Skim milk
Buttermilk
Low-fat yogurt
Low-fat cottage cheese
Mozzarella cheese
Monterey Jack Cheese

Make sure that these milk products are fresh when you buy them; check the date on the package. Eat these milk products in moderation; every other day, for example. Or use them as a security valve when you feel like cheating on your diet. You can add honey and cinnamon to yogurt and cottage cheese, put half a slice of mozzarella on a two-egg garlic omelette when it's about ready to take out of the oven, or make a delicious grilled-cheese sandwich with whole wheat bread. A teaspoon of blackstrap molasses in a warm glass of skim or buttermilk will make a comforting drink once in a while. Use your imagination.

Remember that dairy products are not the wonder foods they were once thought to be, but they still play an essential part in your diet. Their primary inconvenience is too much fat, thus too many calories. The selection of milk products allowed in the regular part of the Cheater's Diet do away with most fat.

As for which drinks are allowed in the Cheater's Diet, there's a whole chapter (21) on the subject.

FOOD SUBSTITUTION

There are two kinds of food substitution. The first is a no-no: the substitution of a natural food for an artificial one that is loaded with chemicals, such as egg substitutes or fruit juice "beverages." Those substitutes may contain less calories or fat but they also endanger your health in the long run. Besides, why pay the price of the real thing for an inferior product?

The other kind of substitution has to do with replacing a good food you don't like for a good food you do like. If you don't like carrots, you don't have to eat them, as long as you live. The same with salad. You can go all your life without eating any salad if you don't like it and you will be perfectly healthy. Instead, you can eat other kinds of vegetables from which your body would find all its nutritive needs. Far up North, the Inuit peoples used to live almost exclusively on a high-fat, high-meat diet, and they were as healthy as anyone, for the colder the climate the more calories you need. Then "civilized" people started bringing them junk foods by plane in exchange for their furs and art works, and soon they too were plagued with heart disease and cancer.

If you don't enjoy meat, you can eat eggs or yogurt and your protein requirement will be met. There's no one single food or no one food group that you must eat on a *regular* everyday basis to be healthy. The human body is a marvel of nature; just give it fresh, natural foods and it will do the rest. The old theory that a well-balanced diet must include two servings of each of the basic four food groups (meat, milk, fruit-vegetable, bread-cereal) every day doesn't hold water. Your body can store vitamins A, D, E, K for months; it can signal you whether your system needs fluids or solids, sweets or salts, protein or vegetables. People adapt to their environment, not the other way around. Do you think cave men and women had two servings of the basic four food groups daily? And do you want to bet they were healthier than we are?

We may live longer today but not necessarily because we are healthier. Simply because medical technology has almost entirely eliminated the natural selection among our species. And we do pay the price in many ways.

FOOD CHART

Following is a general list of allowed and forbidden foods in the Cheater's Diet. Use the chart as a reference. Foods listed in the forbidden column are too high in calories and they are unhealthy.

The Cheater's Diet

Allowed	Forbidden
Almonds	Applesauce
Apricots	Avocado
Apple	Bacon
Apple cider vinegar	Bologna
Apple juice	Beef (any kind)
Artichokes	Bread crumbs
Asparagus	Butter
Bananas	Cakes
Beets	Cereal (regular)
Broccoli	Coconut
Brown rice	Corn (cream style)
Brussels sprouts	Coffee
Buttermilk	Cola
Cantaloupe	Cookies
Cauliflower	Cheese
Carrots	Cranberry juice
Cabbage	Cream
Celery	Dates (dried)
Chicken (skinless)	Dill pickles (and others)
Chives	Doughnuts
Cottage cheese (low-fat)	Figs (dried)
Corn on the cob	Green peas (canned)
Cucumber	Gravy (any kind)
Duck	Ham
Eggplant	Hamburgers
Eggs	Hot dogs
Endive	Ice cream
Fish (fresh, without breadcrumb coating)	Jam
	Ketchup
Grapes	Margarine
Grapefruit juice	Marmalade
Green leaf	Mayonnaise
Honey (unpasteurized)	Milk (regular and evaporated)
Honeydew	Noodles
Kiwi	Oranges
Lamb	Oils

Allowed	Forbidden
Lemon	Pancakes
Lettuce	Pasta
Lime	Popcorn (with butter and salt)
Lima beans (cooked only)	Prune juice
Lean meats	Peanut butter
Lentils (cooked only)	Pecans
Lobster	Pizza
Mangos	Pies
Mozzarella cheese	Potato chips
Mushrooms	Raisins (dried)
Mustard	Relish
Mustard greens	Salad dressing
Nectarines	Salami
Nuts (plain and in small amounts)	Sauces
Oatmeal	Soups
Onions	Sour cream
Parsley	Sugar
Papayas	Syrup
Peaches	Tapioca
Peanuts (plain—unroasted)	Tea
Pineapple	Tuna
Pimiento	White rice
Popcorn (unsalted—unbuttered)	White bread
Potatoes (baked, boiled, or Cheater's potatoes)	White flour products
Pumpkin	Yogurt (whole milk with fruits)
Raspberries	Vinegar
Radishes	
Rhubarb	
Rutabaga	
Shrimp	
Skim milk	
Spinach	
Soybeans (cooked only)	
Strawberries	
Sunflower seeds	

Allowed	Forbidden
Tomatoes	
Tomato juice	
Turkey	
Turnips	
Tuna (packed in water)	
Yogurt (low-fat)	
Watercress	
Watermelon	
Whole wheat bread and crackers	
Wheat germ	
Veal	
Zucchini	

HOW MANY MEALS A DAY?

How many meals a day should you eat while on the Cheater's Diet? You can lose weight eating only once a day and you can lose weight eating five small meals a day. It's a matter of total calorie intake at the end of the day, not of how many meals you've eaten. Five meals a day is impractical, and one big, single meal may be taxing for the digestive system. Therefore, two to four small meals a day would best serve the purpose of most dieters.

Breakfast is regarded by many authorities as the most important meal of the day. This is only partially true. When you wake up in the morning, there's no reason for you to crave food unless you haven't eaten well the day before. Although most people aren't hungry upon arising in the morning, they force themselves to eat something because they think they will fall flat on their faces if they don't. Instead, they should wait half an hour or so and then—*if* they are hungry—eat a little. If they are not hungry, they would do better to wait until lunch time to eat.

On the other hand, your first meal of the day—whether you have it at eight in the morning or one in the afternoon—is important because your stomach is empty. Everything, whether it's food or a drug, is better absorbed by an empty stomach.

As a general rule, don't eat when you're not hungry. If you do, at best you won't lose weight and at worst you'll gain. To reduce your weight you have to keep your body in a *catabolic* state. When you're not hungry your body is telling you it has energy in reserve. Listen to it. You don't need exactly the same amount of calories every day.

When I first tested the Cheater's Diet (for a five-week period), I was eating three small, regular meals a day, plus a low-calorie snack before going to bed. Many years later, it's still the best way for me whether I want to lose weight or just maintain it.

I suggest that you start the Cheater's Diet eating four times a day; you can cut down to three or two meals if it's more practical for you. Make your own adjustments as you go along. Just be careful to start by consuming about 1,000 calories a day.

Warning: Never go under 600 calories a day for prolonged periods of time in an attempt to lose weight faster. Super-low-calorie diets can cause death!

A Regular Eating-Day Sample

BREAKFAST	one of the following
	1 apple
(about 225 calories)	1 egg
	1 whole wheat toast
	OR
	1 bowl of oatmeal with cinnamon and honey
(about 244 calories)	½ banana
	½ cup of pineapple juice
	OR
(about 245 calories)	1 banana sandwich
	½ cup of buttermilk
LUNCH	
	1 chicken breast with brown rice
(about 350 calories)	1 tomato salad
	cucumber
	½ cup of skim milk
	OR
	½ grapefruit
(about 350 calories)	2 egg omelette with mushrooms
	½ cup of low-fat yogurt with ½ teaspoon honey
	OR

(about 320 calories)	1 filet of sole with seasoning 1 baked potato 1 stalk of steamed broccoli 1 medium tomato
DINNER:	
(about 350 calories)	lobster (a small serving) ½ cub brown rice seasoned with lime 1 cup of zucchini
	OR
(about 350 calories)	2 egg garlic-omelette 1 baked potato asparagus (6 spears) 1 nectarine—medium
	OR
(about 350 calories)	lamb (1 small serving) Brussels sprouts (½ cup) 1 baked potato ½ cup apple juice
BEDTIME SNACK	Celery, carrots, or cucumber
	OR
	1 cup of warm skim milk with cinnamon
	OR
	1 egg
	OR
	1 banana
	OR
	1 toast with honey

A GUIDE TO SEASONINGS

Without a doubt, seasonings can make a big difference between a boring diet and an exciting one.

To get maximum enjoyment from your daily foods, they must look good, smell good and above all, they must taste good.

If you add seasoning to a cooked dish, do it when the cooking is almost done so the flavor won't have time to evaporate. On a cold dish, let seasonings impregnate long enough to get maximum flavor. Don't mix too many seasonings in one dish—more often than not, one or two is enough. Though most seasonings listed in the next pages don't contain calories per se, they should be used sparingly for best results.

Remember also that the following list reflects my preferences. Feel free to try any combination that suits your fancy. Who knows what you may discover?

Spices

Cinnamon: Available on the market in powder or small sticks. Use the powder on cereals, apple, veal, potatoes, low-fat cottage cheese, and yogurt. Use sticks in punches or hot beverages (skim and buttermilk).

Mustard: Use the powder with meat, dressing, and egg dishes.

Pepper: Ground pepper can be used with fish, chicken, dressing, and stews. Powder can be used on anything but sweet dishes.

Paprika: Can be employed with eggs, chicken, veal, dressing, and goulash.

Curry Powder: Best utilized with meat, chicken, seafoods, eggs, brown rice, and vegetables. Can also be added sparingly to salad and dressing.

Nutmeg: Sprinkle on all vegetables, especially green, leafy ones. Can be used on most cooked dishes as well.

Cayenne Pepper: Should be used sparingly—with chili con carne, egg dishes, and stews.

Herbs

Mint: Use the leaves to decorate beverages, salads, or fruit dishes. Mint is delicious with carrots and veal. (See the mint-sauce recipe on p. 84—*Minted Carrots*.)

Tarragon: The dry leaves of tarragon can be used sparingly with chicken, lamb, veal, and salads.

Parsley: Use on brown rice, potatoes, omelettes, veal, salads, cottage cheese, and tomato juice.

Thyme: Available in powder or leaves. Thyme has a strong flavor. Use lightly with fish, chicken, turkey, and potatoes.

Oregano: Use with lentils, tomato juice, egg dishes, vegetable stews, and salads.

Basil: Available in powder or leaves. Delicate flavor. Best used with zucchini, tomatoes, carrots, spinach, salads, fish, meat, and seafood.

Sage: Strong flavor. Use sparingly on tomatoes, salads, and veal.

Rosemary: Available in leaves. Special aroma. Use with seafoods, chicken, veal, and vegetables.

Marjoram: Delicate flavor. Powder or leaves. Can be used with most dishes that aren't sweet.

Natural Flavorings

Vanilla: Best used with yogurt, cottage cheese, oatmeal, cream of wheat, and protein drink.

Lime: Adds zest to brown rice, fish, shrimp, lobster, salad and chicken, desserts, and drinks. The subtle flavor and unique perfume of lime will bring a touch of exoticism to any dish.

Lemon: Use mainly with fish and salads but remember: anything lemon can do, lime will do much better.

Almonds: Best served with fruit salads, cereals, and fish (especially sole and yellow pike).

Honey: (unpasteurized) Use sparingly to flavor yogurt, cottage cheese, oatmeal, toast, and lemonade.

Other Seasonings

Pimiento: A good source of natural vitamin C. Chopped pimiento enhances any salad and gives zest to a plain omelette. Can also be added to casseroles or stews.

Apple cider vinegar: Can be used straight from the bottle on all kinds of salads or mixed with other ingredients to make your own favorite dressing.

*Garlic: Fresh garlic is served best with tossed salads, omelettes, seafood, and brown rice.

Capers: Try it with lamb, fish, omelette, and tossed salads.

Chives: Best with potatoes, veal, and cottage cheese.

Shallots: Use with egg dishes, cottage cheese, and salads. Shallots have a lighter taste than onions. You can enjoy the green part as well as the white.

---

*Beware. You can go to jail in Gary, Indiana, for riding on a streetcar less than four hours after eating garlic. It's the law in Gary!

Onion: Stews, casseroles, salads, omelettes, eggs, and many other dishes can benefit from onions as a seasoning. Don't be afraid to do some experimenting.

CHEATER'S DIET RECIPES

Every dieter loves recipes, not necessarily the preparations but certainly the consumption of the final product. In these pages you'll be introduced to a sample of the new cuisine. I hope the dishes presented will convince you that the new trend in cooking is not only low fat calories but also light and tasty.

Any of the following recipes can be used for your regular meals.

The two menus suggested at the end of this chapter should preferably serve as part of a cheating meal, being more elaborate, thus higher in calories, especially if you have a good wine with it, as you should. Try this test. Invite some of your best friends and serve them either the Cheater's Diet Dinner à la carte or the Special Dinner. But wait until the end of the meal to tell them they ate a diet menu, and watch the reactions.

Following is the most important recipe of all. Read it every day until you know it by heart.

Recipe for Losing Weight

3 cups of willingness
3 cups of knowledge (copy of the Cheater's Diet)
½ pound of exercise
½ pound of sacrifice
1 cup of confidence
1 tablespoon of hope
A dash of imagination

Put willingness and knowledge into your lifestyle. Mix slowly with confidence and hope. Add sacrifice and exercise regularly. Sprinkle with imagination.

Cook for two weeks to six months. Season at will.

Main Dishes

du Tremblay Pot-au-Feu

4 ounces vegetable broth
4 cups water
2 pounds veal—1" cubes
2 carrots (diced)

¼ cup turnips (diced)
½ cup celery (diced)
¼ chopped onion
4 medium potatoes
½ cup cabbage
⅛ teaspoon rosemary
¼ teaspoon sage
pepper to taste

In a big stewing pot start cooking the vegetable broth with cold water. At boiling point, add the meat and seasonings. Cover and let simmer two hours. Add the veggies 45 minutes before the end of cooking so they will be done when ready to serve.

Serves 4.

Cheater's Casserole

3 tablespoons chicken broth
1 cup chopped onions
1 teaspoon curry powder
3 tablespoons whole wheat flour
2 cups buttermilk
¼ teaspoon savory
⅛ teaspoon rosemary
Dash of pepper
2 cups cooked French beans
3 cups cooked turkey (cut and diced)
2 tablespoons chopped pimiento
¼ cup chopped almonds

Sauté the onions in the chicken broth until transparent. Then add the curry and cook a few more seconds. Put seasonings and whole wheat flour in the pan and cook while stirring until smooth and thick. Add turkey, French beans, and pimiento. Pour in a Teflon oven pot, cover, and cook for half an hour at 350° F. Then uncover, sprinkle the almonds over the dish, and let cook for ten more minutes.

Serves 6.

Omelette Claudine

2 eggs
1 tablespoon cold water
½ slice mozzarella cheese
parsley
garlic
pimiento

Put eggs and water in a blender and blend for five seconds. Pour in a Teflon cooking pan. Cook at medium heat until nearly done. Then add parsley, chopped fresh garlic, cheese and put in oven at 350° F for five minutes. When ready top off with chopped pimiento.
Serves 1.

Cheater's Brochette

4 tablespoons chicken broth
6 tablespoons low-fat soy sauce
¼ teaspoon ground pepper
1 onion, finely grated
3 tablespoons lime juice
3 pounds veal steak, cut into 1" cubes

Make a marinade with the mixed ingredients. Cut veal into cubes and leave in the marinade for at least one hour, turning and rubbing the seasonings into the meat. Thread on skewers with whole mushrooms, small tomatoes, and pieces of pimiento between the meat. Broil.
Serves 6.

Casserole Amandine

2¼ tablespoons vegetable broth
¾ cup chopped onions
1 teaspoon curry powder
2½ tablespoons whole wheat flour
Dash of pepper
⅛ teaspoon of rosemary
1½ cups buttermilk
1½ cups green beans (cooked)
2½ cups cooked turkey (diced)
1½ tablespoons pimiento
¼ cup almond flakes

Sauté the onions until transparent in the vegetable broth. Add curry and cook 15 seconds. Slowly mix in flour and seasonings. Add milk gradually and cook while stirring until thick and smooth. Add beans, turkey, and pimiento. Pour in a deep non-stick pan. Cover and cook 20 minutes at 375° F. Uncover, garnish with almonds, and cook five more minutes.
Serves 4.

Cheating Con Carne

1½ tablespoons chicken broth
¾ cup chopped onions
1 garlic clove, smashed

1¼ pounds *extra lean* ground beef*
2¼ tablespoons chili powder
⅛ teaspoon pepper
20 ounces canned tomatoes
20 ounces canned red beans

Sauté onions and garlic in chicken broth until transparent. Add beef and cook until browned. Drain excess fat. Mix in seasoning and tomatoes. Cover and simmer for about two hours or until thick. Add beans and cook some more.

Serves 4.

Rice 'n' Nice

½ cup brown rice
2 chopped shallot stalks
1 chopped celery stalk
⅛ cup chopped red pepper
1 cup vegetable juice
3 large mushrooms
Dash of ground pepper

Cook the rice (medium heat) in a nonstick pan until toasted evenly. Add vegetable juice, shallots, celery, red pepper, mushrooms, and pepper. Mix thoroughly. Simmer (covered) until all water has evaporated (about 35 minutes).

Serves 2.

Cheater's Quiche

1 9 in. whole wheat pie crust
4 eggs
1½ cups of buttermilk
⅛ teaspoon tarragon
1 cup cooked shrimps
½ cup grated mozzarella cheese
¼ cup chopped onions and pimiento

Set the oven at 400° F. Partially cook pie crust in oven for about eight minutes. Take out and lower oven to 350° F. Beat eggs slightly. Add buttermilk, pepper, and other seasonings. Cover pie crust with shrimps, cheese, onions, and pimiento. Pour over beaten egg mixture and place in oven for 35 to 40 minutes.

Serves 4 to 6.

---

*Cheating Con Carne is the only dish in which beef is permitted because no other meat will do. So make sure it's extra lean; ask the butcher to prepare it especially for you.

Fillet de Sole Amandine

½ cup lime juice
4 slices fillet of sole
4 tablespoons low-fat yogurt
½ teaspoon parsley flakes
Dash of onion powder
¼ cup almond flakes

Put fillet in a baking dish, cover with lime juice, and let it marinate for an hour or more. Spread the fish with yogurt, onion powder, and parsley. Broil for ten minutes or until cooked to your liking.

Before serving top with almond flakes. Serve with Cheater's mashed potatoes.

Serves 4.

Veal-o-Veggies

2 pounds veal (cubes)
2 onions
3 garlic cloves
5 carrots (round sliced)
3 stalks of celery (diced)
½ green pepper (diced)
1 turnip (diced)
Season with pepper and capers

Add water to make a broth and cook two hours at low heat. Serve with baked potatoes.

Serves 4.

Side Dishes

Minted Carrots

4 large carrots (sliced)
¼ teaspoon dried mint
¼ teaspoon grated lime rind

Cook carrots until nearly done. Then remove excess water, leaving only a small amount of water. Add lime rind and mint. Cover and cook for five more minutes. Drain and serve.

Serves 2.

Stuffed Tomatoes

4 lettuce leaves
4 tomatoes
2 7 oz. cans tuna flakes (packed in water)
1 small green pepper

1 big celery stalk (chopped)
1 small onion (chopped)
⅓ cup apple cider vinegar
pepper
parsley

Remove seeds from pepper and dice. In a bowl mix the tuna, celery, green pepper, apple cider, and pepper. Put in fridge for 15 minutes. Turn tomatoes upside down and with a sharp knife cut them, but not completely, into six parts. Open each tomato gently and throw in a bit of pepper. Top with the tuna mixture and sprinkle lightly with parsley. Serve the tomatoes on a lettuce leaf on individual platters.

Aspic-o-Veggies

1 cup of carrots (diced)
1 cup of celery cut in small pieces
1 cup of low-fat yogurt (plain)
3 ounces unflavored gelatin
1 tablespoon of lime juice
¾ cup boiling water

Dissolve gelatin in boiling water with lime and wait until it thickens. When gelatin is consistent enough, add carrots, celery, yogurt, and mix slowly. When ready to serve, flip over a salad and decorate.

Cheaters' Potatoes

buttermilk
parsley (fresh or dried flakes)
egg whites
onion powder
dash of pepper (optional)

Peel and cook potatoes in water, as usual. Drain hot water and add one or two egg whites, mash the potatoes, cover, and wait 30 seconds. Then add some buttermilk, onion powder, and parsley. Mash again. Serve with meat, fish, or poultry.

Asparagus du Tremblay

1 bunch fresh asparagus
du Tremblay *special* dressing (see p. 87)

Cook asparagus until tender. Remove from water and set on a platter. Pour some du Tremblay special dressing over the dish to suit your taste.

Brussels Sprouts Royal

1 pound fresh Brussels sprouts
¼ cup lime juice

¼ teaspoon onion powder
⅛ teaspoon dry mustard

Cook sprouts until tender. Put in a serving dish. Mix the lime juice, mustard, and onion powder; pour sauce over the vegetable and serve.

Cabbage Fruit Salad

4 cups grated green cabbage
1 cup pineapple (diced)
1 cup diced red apple
½ cup chopped celery

Gently mix the ingredients. Add ¾ cup of du Tremblay special dressing (without garlic) to which you have previously mixed two tablespoons of pineapple juice.

Exotic Fruit Salad

20 oz. low-fat plain yogurt
1 teaspoon apple cider vinegar
½ cup chopped almonds
1 pineapple (diced)
3 sliced bananas

Mix the first three ingredients, and then add the other two. Mix well. Refrigerate for at least two hours. Add red cherries before serving.

Fiesta Salad

½ head romaine lettuce
2 shallot sticks
⅛ cup apple cider vinegar
1 tablespoon lime juice
1 tablespoon water
⅛ teaspoon dry mustard
pepper to taste

Tear the salad into pieces, put it in a bowl, and add the chopped shallots. Mix remaining ingredients together and pour over the salad. Toss and serve.

Dressing and Sauces

Three Star Dressing

½ cup tomato juice
2 tablespoons low-fat yogurt (plain)
1 tablespoon lime juice
¼ teaspoon onion powder

Put the ingredients in a blender and mix at low speed for five seconds, and it's ready to serve.

Dressing du Chef

¼ cup lime juice
¼ cup cider vinegar
¼ cup apple juice
½ teaspoon garlic powder
¼ teaspoon dry mustard

    Mix well and serve.

Hot Potato Sauce

⅔ cup low-fat plain yogurt
2 tablespoons prepared mustard
2 tablespoons capers
1 tablespoon lime juice

    Yields one cup.

du Tremblay Special Dressing

½ cup apple cider vinegar
¼ cup low-fat plain yogurt
1 tablespoon fresh lime juice
fresh garlic to taste

    Mix well and serve.

Cheaters' Sauce

1⅓ cups of non-fat plain yogurt
⅓ cup chili sauce
¼ cup mustard
¼ cup chopped onions
½ teaspoon of parsley
⅛ teaspoon cayenne pepper

    Sieve the chile sauce for a smoother texture. Then mix all the ingredients in a bowl. Beat with a fork to get an even mix. Keep sauce in refrigerator for a few hours before serving. Serve hot or cold with fish, turkey, chicken, and veal.

    Yields about two cups.

Francis' Dressing

¾ cup apple cider vinegar
¼ cup lime juice
1¼ tablespoons mustard
1¼ tablespoons tomato purée
1 teaspoon onion powder
¼ teaspoon celery powder
½ teaspoon paprika
dash of black pepper

Put the ingredients in a bottle and shake until you get a perfect mixture. Always shake well before serving.

Shrimp Sauce

1 cup tomato juice
1 tablespoon apple cider vinegar
2 tablespoons lime juice
1 teaspoon grated shallots
¼ teaspoon dry mustard
⅛ teaspoon garlic powder

Mix the ingredients thoroughly in a tightly closed bottle. Serve sauce on the side with shrimps or clams.

Asparagus Sauce

4 tablespoons low-fat plain yogurt
4 teaspoons lime juice
4 teaspoons prepared mustard

Yields 4 servings.

Red Baron Dressing

½ cup cider vinegar
½ cup tomato juice
1½ tablespoons lime juice
¼ teaspoon garlic powder
¾ tablespoon chopped shallots
pepper and paprika to taste

Breakfasts

Cheap-Grocery-Breakfast Drink

10 ounces pineapple juice
1 tablespoon wheat germ
2 tablespoons protein powder*
1 egg yolk
½ banana

Cheap-Grocery Breakfast

2 eggs (hard, soft boiled, or poached)
1 toast
½ banana
½ cup skim milk

---

*Milk and egg protein powder is best. Soya protein is too high in calories, harder to digest when eaten raw, and has a lower P.E.R. (Protein Efficiency Ratio). Take note, however, that soya can yield twice as much protein value when cooked properly; that is, 140°F for three minutes.

Try eating one of these two breakfasts ½ hour to 1 hour before doing your groceries. It's the secret to buying only the food you had on your list and nothing extra. You'll be amazed at the money you will save in the long run and how much easier it will be to follow your diet.

Note: If you work from 9 to 5, buy your groceries on the weekend. It's wiser to do your shopping in the morning when you're fresh and when the supermarket is not so crowded. You can thus avoid impulsive buying.

Breakfast of Champions

2 eggs
1 tablespoon water
6 large strawberries
½ ripe banana
1 teaspoon pure honey
dash of cinnamon

Put the eggs and water in a blender. Mix for 5 seconds. Cook omelette on the stove in a nonstick pan. While omelette is cooking put the strawberries, honey, and banana in blender and mix into a purée.

When the omelette is ready, put it in a serving platter; pour the purée on one half of omelette and fold other half over. Sprinkle with cinnamon.

Serves 1 (about 275 calories).

Cottage à la Mode

4–6 ounces low-fat cottage cheese
1 slice of pineapple
1 teaspoon of unpasteurized honey
dash of cinnamon

Mix honey into the cheese, top with pineapple, and sprinkle with cinnamon.

Serves 1.

French Toast à la Tremblay

½ banana
⅓ teaspoon vanilla extract
1 egg
½ cup buttermilk
2 slices of whole wheat bread
2 teaspoons of honey
cinnamon

Put the egg, milk and vanilla in a blender. Mix for fifteen seconds. Dip bread in the batter and cook in a non-stick pan. Cover each toast with honey and sliced banana. Sprinkle with cinnamon.

Serves 1.

Note: ½ cup of skim milk or juice is allowed with this meal.

Cheaters' Mini-Breakfast

1 egg yolk
1 cup of pineapple juice
1 tablespoon wheat germ
1 teaspoon honey

> Put ingredients in a blender. Mix for fifteen seconds.
> Serves 1 (about 200 calories).

Sure-Cure Hangover Breakfast*

10 oz. unsweetened apple juice
3 tablespoons protein powder
1 teaspoon wheat germ
1 kiwi fruit

> Peel the kiwi and mix with other ingredients in a blender for 10 seconds. Drink slowly and imbue each sip thoroughly with saliva for better digestion.

Cinnamon Oatmeal

1 cup large flakes oatmeal
2 tablespoons protein powder
½ teaspoon cinnamon

> Mix the ingredients in a bowl. Bring two and a half cups of water to boiling point and pour the dry mixture into it. Cook a few minutes while stirring.
> Top with sliced banana and one tablespoon of honey.
> Serves 2.

Oven-Warm Breakfast

2 slices whole wheat bread
1 tomato
1 slice mozzarella cheese
pepper

> Cover the bread with ½ slice mozzarella cheese. Top with sliced tomatoes, add a dash of pepper, and put in the oven (350° F) until cheese is melted. Serve at once.
> You can add to this breakfast ½ cup of skim milk or any allowed juice.
> Yields about 350 calories.
> Serves 1.

---

*If you want to avoid a hangover after a big party, drink 2–3 *tall* glasses of water as soon as you come home. You'll be fresh as a rose in the morning—guaranteed. In case you forget or you don't like water, have the Sure-Cure Hangover Breakfast as your first meal of the day.

The reason for a hangover is dehydration due to too much alcohol.

Desserts and Drinks

Omelette Soufflé à la vanille

4 eggs
¾ teaspoon vanilla extract
2 tablespoons cold water
1 tablespoon whole wheat flour
1 tablespoon honey

Beat the egg yolks (with vanilla and honey) until frothy; add the cold water and flour.

Whip egg whites into soft peaks and mix lightly with the yolks. Pour in a nonstick pan and cook in the oven for 20 minutes at 350° F. Don't open the oven during cooking or your soufflé will flatten.

Yields about 200 calories per serving.
Serves 2.

Strawberry Surprise

2 cups fresh strawberries
½ cup papaya juice
½ cup low-fat vanilla yogurt
1 tablespoon undiluted frozen apple juice

Hull the strawberries and put them in a bowl. Add the papaya juice and toss. Top the dish with yogurt mixed with apple juice.

Serves 2.

Tropical Punch

30 ounces low-fat vanilla yogurt
12 ounces pineapple juice
4 ounces papaya juice
1 tablespoon fresh lime juice
16 ounces buttermilk

Blend the ingredients thoroughly in an electric mixer. Serve with crushed ice.

Serves about 10.

Summer Party Punch

36 ounces of papaya juice
48 ounces grapefruit juice
48 ounces pineapple juice
30 ounces cold water
juice of 3 limes
3 trays of ice cubes

Decorate with lime wedges and red cherries.
Serves 30.

P.S. If you're at the legal drinking age in your state, you can add a bottle of rum to this recipe.

Grape Punch

2 cups grape juice
1 cup apple juice
juice of 1 lime
2 cups cold water
4 tablespoons honey

Mix well and refrigerate for 24 hours.
Serves 6.

Cheater's Special Dinner
MENU

Entrée:	Shrimp cocktail with shrimp sauce
Salad:	Fiesta Salad
Main Dish:	Cheater's Brochette served on garlic brown rice
Side Dish:	Brussels Sprouts Royal
Dessert:	Strawberry Surprise

Cheater's Dinner à la Carte
MENU

Entrée:	Stuffed Tomatoes
Salad:	Roman Salad with du Tremblay Special Dressing
Main Dish:	Fillet de Sole Amandine served with Cheaters' Potatoes
Side Dish:	Minted Carrots
Dessert:	Omelette Soufflé à la vanille

ENJOY YOUR MEAL

19

WHY CHEATING IS A MUST

Variety's the very spice of life, that gives it all its flavor. (William Cowper)

A famous artist once said: "I use to sit down in front of an appetizing dessert of strawberry pie and whipped cream to see if I could resist the temptation of eating it. Then, when I was absolutely sure I could, I ate it to reward myself."

Herein lies the foundation and philosophy of the Cheater's Diet. Behaviorism stresses the role of environment as a determinant of human behavior; in regard to the eating patterns of the American people, this has never been truer than today. When one is solicited, brainwashed, and programmed by food publicity 24 hours a day, it's almost impossible not to be influenced by such an environment.

How many times have you been tempted by the junk food devil with the promise of a joyous feast only to realize you had been lured into gastronomic folly with laborious digestion as your sole reward? Temptation can be resisted but not always. With the Cheater's Diet you can have your cake and eat it too; every four days, you reward yourself with a scheduled everything-goes meal (cheating meal) because you have faithfully followed the regular part of the diet.

THE HEART OF THE DIET

Cheating meals are the heart of the Cheater's Diet. Cheating is necessary because most diets fail in the short run and all diets fail in the long run. *All* who read this book, cheat on their diets. Don't tell me it isn't so because, otherwise, you'd be at your normal weight, and you feel guilty as well. And you cheat more and more until, discouraged, you drop a diet entirely and go on an eating binge thinking you are destined to be fat and unhappy forever.

You could save yourself all this trouble when you understand that cheating is a matter of knowing when and how to cheat, as you will learn in this chapter.

But first you have to throw away all the standard ideas about dieting. You have to accept the concept that cheating once in a while is not bad for you and that it will actually speed up your progress.

Even with regular cheating meals, the Cheater's Diet is definitely a quality diet. Theoretically, an ideal diet has a 100 percent quality factor. But because of the way food is grown and processed, and because of additives, pesticides, colorants, and storage, no diet can pretend to such a quality level. I estimate the quality factor of the Cheater's Diet to be at the top of the scale—about 90 percent—because it allows you to eat fresh fruits, fresh vegetables, lean meat, eggs, fish, nuts, whole wheat bread, and cereal. The regular part of the Cheater's Diet is essentially low in fat and free of junk foods. The only food group excluded on a regular basis is that of dairy products, which are not intended by nature for adult consumption anyway.

Cheating meals occur at the frequency of one in every fifteen regular meals (if you eat three meals a day), and 1/15 of 90 percent equals 6 percent; thus we arrive at a staggering 84 percent quality factor. How does the average American diet rate in comparison? I can tell you it's in the neighborhood of 50 percent and most popular diets today don't have more than a 60 percent quality factor.

As you can see the Cheater's Diet is a quality program. But why cheat at all? Wouldn't it be better to skip the cheating part if you had enough willpower to do so? The answer is no. When you go on a low-calorie diet you lose weight at first, and then you usually reach a plateau due to the fact that your system burns up calories at a slower rate as a survival mechanism. But, by throwing in a cheating meal every now and then (between the low-calorie days), you *fool your body* into thinking you're not on a diet. It doesn't know what to expect and you end up the winner.

WINNING OVER FRUSTRATION

Probably the biggest advantage for you in cheating is that it prevents the build up of frustration over your favorite foods. Let's face it, everyone has a weakness for certain foods that happen to have a high caloric content. Mine is warm chocolate chip cookies and strawberry cheesecake. (Now you know everything about me.)

One reason most diets fail is because they never give you a break. They don't take into account the human factor. They don't talk about cheating, presuming everyone is endowed with superhuman willpower; if they talk about it at all, they only suggest that cheating is an evil you have to contend with the best you can.

Why Cheating's a Must

The bottom line of *any* long-term project is sustained motivation. Fortunately, the Cheater's Diet is designed with today's life-style in mind. One cheating meal every four days will prevent long-term frustration. But what about short-term frustration? What do you do if you find yourself craving your favorite food two days after you had a cheating meal?

There are two techniques that can solve that problem.

1. Lie down on the living room couch or on your bed (the place must be quiet) and close your eyes. Relax as much as you can. Then, by self-suggestion, persuade yourself that if you wait two more days for the scheduled cheating meal, your pleasure will be more intense, beyond anything you could expect if you cheated now.

Visualize yourself eating your favorite food on the scheduled cheating meal, picture the amount you will have, how each bite will taste, how much greater your satisfaction will be because you haven't failed. Then, when you feel in control of your hunger, get up and drink a tall glass of water or eat a few stalks of celery and resume your activities.

2. Try to do manual work that requires some skill and attention. Repair that flat on your bike, fix the leaky sink, mow the lawn, do the Cube, or anything else you can think of. You also can do real physical exertion: push-ups, deep knee bends, jogging, socking the punching bag in the basement, swimming if you've got a pool, or simply walk. Exercise stimulates the production of hormones, cutting down your hunger for a while; besides, it relaxes you and you feel (and are) more in control of your emotions.

Yet, human nature being what it is, we must consider the eventuality of failure. What should you do if you cheat in the four days of regular or straight eating? You start anew and schedule your next cheating meal four days later. For example, let's say you had a cheating meal on Monday. This means your next cheating meal is scheduled on Saturday. But Thursday night you are unable to resist that strawberry cheesecake (I knew I wasn't alone) and now you're wondering what to do. Simply start over again and schedule your next cheating meal four days later; that is, next Tuesday. Then promise yourself that the next time you will be the winner.

Warning: The four-day lapse between each scheduled cheating meal is not an arbitrary period of time. It's to ensure a maximum weight loss with minimum food frustration. Under no circumstances should you depart from this four-day rule (the cornerstone of the Cheater's Diet) or you will defeat the purpose of the program. The only exception to this rule is explained in Chapter 22.

20

HOW TO CHEAT EFFECTIVELY

Every guilty person is his own hangman. (Seneca)

"Guilty, your Honor," said the delinquent.
"Of what?" asked the judge, puzzled. "You haven't been accused yet."
"I've been cheating on my diet for the past two months, your Honor."
"And what happened?"
"Well, I've lost 24 pounds," said the man. "But somehow I feel guilty of wrongdoing."
"Have you hurt anyone in the process?" asked the judge.
"No, your Honor."
"Well, case dismissed—go away, young man," ordered the judge. Then looking up at the ceiling he said to himself,
"This man can't be anything but innocent."

Guilty and *cheating* are two words that have often been associated. Many people seem unable to relish the sweetness of success when it comes without feeling guilty.

Most of us cheat on our diets, and whether you stick with the Cheater's Diet or not, you will probably cheat for the rest of your life. So why feel guilty? You'd better get used to cheating since you'll have to *live* with it.

THE BEST TIME TO CHEAT

After many experiments with the Cheater's Diet, I've found out that cheating meals are most effective at lunch time and dinner. Cheating before bedtime and at breakfast is not recommended for several reasons. Your ability to enjoy food is at a peak at lunch and dinner time. Cheating on an empty stomach is unhealthy, and gulping down 1,500 calories just before going to bed may not be very healthy either. If you've been dying to have breakfast at your favorite fast-food place and it has turned into an obsession, go ahead and enjoy yourself. The same for that midnight pizza craving. But as a rule, try to plan your cheating sessions for lunch or dinner.

HOW TO CHEAT EFFECTIVELY

Try to finish your cheating meal within half an hour; in a two- or three-hour cheating meal, you could easily cram in 2,000 or 3,000 calories. This would definitely slow your progress if done on a regular basis. The purpose of a cheating meal is to prevent the buildup of food frustration. It's not a busting-out affair. You eat whatever you like until you feel pleasantly full and then you stop. If, after a cheating meal, you feel uncomfortable and bloated—if you have to loosen your belt a few notches, you have not yet mastered the art of cheating. A cheating meal is not a contest to see how many calories you can gulp down in one sitting. Its purpose is to give you a break from the regular part of the diet and to pep you up for another four days of straight dieting. So without counting calories at each cheating meal try to stay under 1,500 calories; that's more than four times the caloric intake of the regular meals you'll be eating on the straight part of the Cheater's Diet.

Once you have reached your desired weight, you can raise the caloric intake of your regular meals. But don't count calories; instead, add a little more of everything and make sure you do it progressively. If you find your weight going up, cut down on your regular eating meals. But don't eliminate a particular food; just cut down on every food you normally eat.

HOW TO AVOID STALENESS

A few months after you've followed the Cheater's Diet and lost many pounds of fat, you may find that you have reached a plateau. The main reason may be that your initial enthusiasm has faded and you have relaxed on your eating too much. At this point, you must reduce the caloric intake of your regular meals. Another reason may be that you are one of those incredible eaters who can easily consume 2,000 calories in less than fifteen minutes. Check the caloric content of one cheating meal to see if this is so. If it is, cut down to about 1,100 calories. Reduction of food intake is the secret to getting out of your rut.

Another explanation for leveling off may be that you have an exceptionally slow metabolism. If you suspect that this is so, try one cheating meal every five days instead of the recommended four. Also cheat with moderation most of the time.

Another reason you're not losing weight might be that you failed too often to respect the four days of regular eating; that is, you may be cheating when you're not supposed to. That's bad. The solution is to avoid no-contest situations. For example, if there's a fast-food place near your home and each day when you pass it you can't help entering and devouring a dozen goodies, change your route. You can still go in that direction every four days.

The following list is a "Junk Food Guide." It's only a sample to give you an idea of which foods are bad and which are even worse. If you have a choice between two junk foods, you may want to choose the lesser of two evils. The food listed in the *Worst* column is not necessarily so because of a higher caloric content but because they rate far lower in overall quality.

THE CHEATER'S GUIDE TO JUNK FOOD

Bad	*Worst*
Apple pie	Chocolate pie
Applesauce (canned)	White sauce
Cookies	Chocolate sauce
Ice cream	Potato chips
Fruitcake	Chocolate cake (with icing)
Fruit cocktail (canned)	Candy bar
Grilled cheese	French fries
Hamburger	Hot dog
Ham	Bacon
Italian dressing oil	Mayonnaise
Jelly	Chocolate pudding
Jam	Processed cheese
Macroni	Salami
Maple syrup	White sugar
Olive oil	Margarine
Pancakes	Jelly-filled doughnuts
Pork	Pepperoni
Fried chicken	Pizza
Relish	Ketchup
Soups	Bologna
Spaghetti	Onion rings
Sherbet	Custard
Tapioca	Sour cream
Tomato sauce	Barbecue sauce
Uncola	Cola
Vanilla ice cream	Chocolate ice cream
White rice	White bread

21

ALL ABOUT DRINKS

He is richest who is content with the least, for content is the wealth of nature. (Socrates)

What you drink is as important as *what you eat* in your quest for healthy, normal body weight. Your body is made up of 70 percent fluid (water) and it's *faster* and *easier* to drink calories than to eat them. Furthermore, beverages in general are the biggest stomach stretchers you can find anywhere. All those bloated beer bellies you see in taverns are the best proof of that.

A young but, alas, very fat girl I once knew was in the habit of drinking 12 to 15 pops a day. I convinced her to substitute water for the colas. Twenty days after the switch, she was 14 pounds lighter; being short in stature, this weight loss made a dramatic improvement in her figure. Of course, she was delighted.

Still, liquids are an important part of nutrition, for while you can go a month or so without eating any food, you cannot live more than a few days without liquids.

The only liquids allowed on the regular or straight part of the Cheater's Diet are the following:

Water
Apple juice
Papaya juice
Grapefruit juice
Pineapple juice
Tomato juice and other vegetable juices
Skim milk
Buttermilk

As for the amount you are allowed to drink (except for water between meals), you must restrict your fluid intake at meal time to about four ounces or half a cup. Of course all the juices listed must be unsweetened. If you have a juicer, make your own vegetable and fruit juice, which are far more nutritious. If you don't have a juicer, try to buy bottled juice instead of frozen or canned juice, for these are too high in sodium. The only thing you can add to those beverages is blackstrap molasses as a supplement but only at breakfast—one teaspoonful, no more. If you can't stand the idea of not drinking coffee in the morning, try this substitute. Bring four ounces of skim milk to a boiling point, pour in a cup, and add a teaspoonful of blackstrap molasses. You'll be surprised how good it tastes.

There are two reasons for restricting your liquid intake with meals to half a cup: first, it sets a limit on your calorie intake and second, it prevents stretching of the stomach.

A LOOK AT THE VILLAINS

Alcoholic beverages lead the way by far as the main villain. Hard liquor is a poison, a killer, and it's a concentrated source of calories—which you cannot afford as a dieter.

Beer and wine, having much less alcohol, are not as bad as hard liquor. However, you're better off without beer or wine because they contain extra calories and they increase your appetite, especially when taken before meals. Treat alcohol like dessert and fast food and have them only with scheduled cheating meals.

Soft drinks have no nutritional value. They are loaded with sugar (12 ounces have the carbohydrate equivalence of five teaspoonfuls of refined sugar) and they contain chemicals such as citric acid and caffeine. Colas are the worst. Many years ago, after colas had popped up on the market like mushrooms after a warm rain, one of my uncles started drinking the stuff at the rate of about 24 bottles a day. And even though he was a teetotaler, he died from cirrhosis of the liver some years later at the age of 47.

Coffee—the great American fix—acts as a drug in your body because the caffeine in it *is* a drug. Because coffee is a stimulant of the central nervous system, many overtired and undernourished people think they can't do without it. But they pay a price for their habit—insomnia, headaches, digestion problems, high blood pressure, etc. Tea, cola, and chocolate also contain significant amounts of caffeine.

Tea, besides containing caffeine, has another poison known as tannic acid, which can cause liver damage. Although tea and coffee do not have calories, they act as a stimulant on your system and upset your digestive processes; two good reasons for a dieter to avoid them. In case you think that switching from regular tea to herbal tea is wise, let me tell you it is not. It's like switching from a regular brand of cigarettes to a low-tar brand. Any kind of smoke is bad for you. Likewise, for any kind of tea. Although some herbal teas have no tannic acid, they do have other toxic substances, which you don't need in your diet.

NO SOUP, THANK YOU

Soup is a liquid food, we all know that, but how many of you know that a regular bowl of soup contains about 12 ounces of greasy stuff? Soup is definitely banned from the Cheater's Diet and the reasons are numerous. Soup is made with almost anything: fatty meat, fish, milk, cream, vegetables, etc. And as a Cheater-Dieter your goal is not to put anything or everything into your body—just some of the time, meaning only on scheduled cheating meals. For a dieter, soup has more drawbacks than any other food I know of. Soups are greasy, they bloat you up, they are not nutritional (because they are overcooked and usually made with leftovers), they take the place of nutritious foods, and they are too high in sodium (and that's not speaking of the salt added to them); and too much sodium retains water in the body. So if you want to avoid the puffy look, stay away from soups.

THE ELIXIR OF LIFE

Water is the true elixir of life, the fountain of youth (delays wrinkles' formation) and the only real thirst-quencher. Yes, I'm talking about good old, plain tap water. By the way, don't buy carbonated water or mineral water (most of them are poorly balanced in minerals); they're a waste of money. But if your tap water has a dubious smell or taste, or if you know for sure it's fluorinated, you should consider buying bottled spring water.

Pure water is a blessing for dieters, since it's free of calories. Unlike some juices that have too much acid, water is neutral. It is the second most important nutrient needed to maintain life (the first being air). Water also helps with digestion and cleans the body of waste products. Above all, water is free. That's probably the main reason it's underestimated.

How much water do you need daily? You should drink water only when you feel like it and as much as you need to satisfy your thirst. Forget the silly advice about drinking eight, ten or twelve glasses a day. There are many factors involved in determining how much water you should drink, such as age, activities, weather, food intake, and the general condition of your health.

As for drinking juice, there's no fixed rule that says you have to drink half a cup of juice after each meal. Many times, a few sips of cool water at the end of a meal will do just as well.

As you have noted, not all juices are allowed in the Cheater's Diet. Prune juice, cranberry juice, grape juice, and others are too high in calories. Orange juice is loaded with chemicals. Lemon juice has too much acid (as much acid as a car battery) and should preferably be used as a food seasoning. Some dentists believe that lemon juice erodes the enamel in teeth.

Skim milk and buttermilk are permitted because they are low in calories and they add variety to the diet.

There's no reason why you shouldn't drink with meals as long as you don't drink too much (no more than half a cup) and as long as you don't drink the wrong kind of liquids (coffee, colas, wine) which can upset your digestion.

If you have a dog, try this experiment. Offer him a bowl of water and a bowl of food at the same time. In most cases he will either drink all he can and won't eat or he will eat first and drink only a small amount. There's a lot to learn from animals; they are not wiser than us but their instincts are still intact.

Note: Not drinking enough water for your body needs can be a cause of cellulite even with women of normal body weight. Other causes of cellulite are eating junk food regularly, lack of exercise, and smoking, as we will see in the next chapter.

22

"SMOKING" CELLULITE AWAY

Much smoking kills live men and cures dead swine. (George D. Prentice)

Many believe that God would have created humans with a chimney had He wanted us to smoke. Corny? Not at all—it makes sense.

I first smoked a cigarette when I was about nine or ten years old. Hiding behind my father's garage, I puffed on the cigarette as I had seen Bogart do on television many times. That first encounter with tobacco made me throw up. Later, when I tried it again, I didn't inhale the smoke but pretended to do so to look tough in front of my buddies.

Around that time, when I was thinking about my future I always saw myself sitting at a typewriter, a cigarette hanging nonchalantly from my lips. Now, more than twenty years later, I can't stand the idea of typing (I write in long hand) and I haven't smoked since.

Why smoke at all?

There are many reasons. Let's have a look at some of them.

1. You want to impress your friends and others, but you can't think of anything more clever to do.
2. You like to have some of your fingers stained a deep brown color that doesn't go away no matter how often you wash.
3. You like starting your day coughing for half an hour and, anyway, you don't like to talk in the morning.
4. You don't know what to do with your money so you couldn't care less about letting $500 to $1,000 a year fly up in smoke.
5. You don't like to socialize and make friends so you keep your bad breath as a protection for your privacy.
6. The quality of your sexual relations is not important to you. (Maybe it is to someone else.)
7. You don't mind having wrinkles prematurely.
8. You think that heartburn has nothing to do with smoking.
9. You find cellulite a good topic of conversation at the beach.
10. You don't mind dying prematurely of lung cancer.

I could go on like this for pages but I won't because this is not a horror book; this is a book about dieting and general health.

SMOKING AND CELLULITE

I didn't find the word *cellulite* in any of my dictionaries and I have a few. Doesn't that tell you something?

Cellulite, or the pathological condition the word implies, doesn't exist. It's a *myth*, developed by money-hungry people.

Biopsies done on "cellulite" show it has the same chemical structure as regular fat cells. So why do pseudo-experts on reducing write books on cellulite describing more than a dozen cellulitis conditions and as many different ways to treat them?

The reason is money. The only thing these people want to reduce is the content of your wallet. Granted, the condition referred to as cellulite has special, orange-skin look, but what do you expect from a body part saturated with fat?

Women are affected by cellulite; men are not. There is a hormonal difference and a specific make-up of fat cells in women. Body parts usually affected by cellulite are the back and sides of the thighs, the buttocks, and sometimes, the back of the upper arms or triceps.

In short, the condition referred to as cellulite is not pathological. It's nothing else but compressed, saturated, unhealthy fat; and it should be treated like any undesirable fat.

Smoking destroys vitamin C in your body. Indeed only three cigarettes a day destroys more than the Minimum Daily Requirement, which is 60 milligrams. One of the functions of vitamin C is to help the body resist infection and another is to protect the circulatory system from fat deposits. So regardless of your weight, if you smoke one or more packs a day and eat junk food regularly, the connection between smoking and cellulite should be evident to anyone. Cellulite is the price a society pays when overconsumption is the rule. Cellulite is not a problem in the Third World where poor people eat little more than the powdered skim milk we send them. This for the simple reason that they have no fat on their bodies; and wherever you find cellulite, you find fat. But wherever you find fat, you don't necessarily find cellulite; your body needs a certain amount of fat to function properly.

So if you want to get rid of cellulite, forget about miracle cures; there aren't any. You have to start eating right (according to the Cheater's Diet). You must also do specific exercises (body building) for the affected body parts. Make sure you drink enough water and stop smoking. In a matter of a few months you will be impressed with the results.

Now you may say, that's fine but how in the world am I going to stop smoking?

Simple. As someone said: "To stop smoking is the easiest thing in the world, I've done it hundreds of times." Joking aside, there is an easy way to kick this bad habit. As soon as you stop smoking, exercise vigorously at least three times a week. Body building and jogging serve this purpose perfectly. Such activities, by producing hormonal secretions and significantly accelerating your blood circulation, will put you in a euphoric state familiar to all physical buffs. And this feeling stays with you for hours after a training session. You will feel relaxed as never before and you'll be able to tolerate the nicotine withdrawal symptoms that occur most strongly in the first two weeks.

Also, reduce your meat consumption and eat more vegetables and fruits. This will decrease the acidity in your body. Research indicates that a more alkaline body lessens the need for nicotine.

And don't try the tapering-off approach. Doing so indicates that you have not *really* decided to stop smoking.

If you follow this advice, not only will you succeed in kicking the habit, but you also won't have to worry about gaining extra pounds. The fact that you have stopped smoking has nothing to do with gaining weight, not directly anyway. The loss of control resulting from withdrawal of nicotine and the fact that the ex-smoker's taste is rejuvenated (because his tongue is not clogged up with tar and nicotine anymore) are the main reasons for this common problem.

But again, exercise and eating the right foods will help you resolve both problems in one shot.

Quit smoking! You can do it if you really want to.

23

THE MODIFIED CHEATER'S DIET

Eat, drink and be merry, for tomorrow ye diet. (William Gilmore Beyner)

The Cheater's Diet, being as versatile as it is efficient, can be modified to accommodate your specific needs. But those alterations shouldn't be made at random; definite rules should be followed.

Why modify the Cheater's Diet at all? There are many reasons. You may want more variety in your diet; or you may be one of those overachievers who wants faster results. What if you end up in the hospital for a month? What should you do about your diet? And what if you have food allergies? Don't worry. The Modified Cheater's Diet will take care of these and other problems.

BASIC ALTERATIONS

In the Cheater's Diet, the only way you can modify the number of days between your cheating meals is by adding more days between such meals. A four-day hiatus between each cheating binge is a minimum. Anything below four days of straight dieting and you will F-A-I-L. On the other hand, you can extend your cheating meals to once every ten days, if you like. But if you do, you cannot take a full day of cheating to compensate for waiting. Unlike other diets, you cannot afford *more than one* cheating meal in a row, for physiological and psychological reasons. A full day (three meals) of cheating is definitely out.

Let's take an example of such an alteration in the Cheater's Diet. Jennifer is a nurse. She works on a ten-day on, five-day off schedule. Jennifer doesn't like to have a cheating meal during the ten days she works; she feels guilty when she does. Besides, in two months she's going to Europe with her sister and she wants to be rid of her fat (she is now thirty pounds overweight). What Jennifer can do is alter her diet to enjoy a cheating meal once every ten days. Then her cheating schedule will fit perfectly with her working schedule. She will lose pounds faster and feel less guilty.

Or, take the case of Jack. He plays curling every Friday night. After the game, he ends up at a pizza place with the guys. He eats huge amounts of the stuff and washes it down with a few beers. Jack is a pizza addict; he wouldn't miss this Friday night binge for anything in the world. But the rest of the week he controls his eating habits quite well. So it would be more practical for Jack to have a cheating meal only once every six days.

As you can see, you can modify the Cheater's Diet to suit your goal or schedule, as long as you have *at least* four days between binges and your cheating binge is limited to only one meal. As a bonus, if you have one cheating meal every six or ten days, you can eat more calories at the meal without compromising your diet.

FOOD ALLERGIES

Many people are allergic to certain foods—even natural, wholesome foods like tomatoes or strawberries. If you are among the unfortunate ones plagued with this problem or if you suspect you might be, the best thing to do is to consult your doctor. Tell him you want to follow the Cheater's Diet and tell him how it works. He may give you permission to indulge in allergic foods once every four days or once every ten days, depending on the food in question and whether it's a minor or major cause of allergies. In any event, because the Cheater's Diet is a balanced nutritional program, your doctor can approve a modified version of it if you have allergies, or if you have diabetes or any other disease.

HOSPITALS

Hospitals are among the worst places to eat, let alone follow the Cheater's Diet adequately. That is understandable. Food budgets in hospitals are generally too low and they are often overcrowded.

So how do you handle a diet if you find yourself confined to a hospital bed for weeks or months?

If you're hospitalized for any appreciable length of time, chances are you are quite sick, and thus are not very hungry; and when you're lying in a hospital bed all day, you don't burn up too many calories. So rule number one of the Modified Cheater's Diet is: Cheating is not allowed in hospitals. Rule number two: Forget about your weight. Think about your *health*. Eat meat, potatoes, and vegetables. Ask friends to bring you fresh fruit, if possible. For some reason there is not enough *fresh* fruit in hospitals. They prefer to give you jello and pudding (junk food). *Don't* touch the stuff. Also don't put poison like coffee or tea in your body when you are *already* sick. Eat only when you're hungry, eat no junk food, drink only water, and *will* yourself to get out of there as soon as possible. Only the body heals but the mind dictates the healing.

MEAL SUBSTITUTES

Here's a list of some delicious, low-calorie (but high-energy) milkshake drinks that you can use once in a while as meal substitutes. They add a welcome variety to the Cheater's Diet. Since these are liquid meals, they are fast to prepare (nothing to cook) and easy to digest. These drinks have nothing to do with the meal substitutes you buy at the drug store, which are expensive and unhealthy. *Note*: I wouldn't recommend that anyone live exclusively on a liquid diet (no matter which one) for more than a month at a time. Your teeth and gums need exercise and your stomach needs more fiber (cellulose) to function properly.

Vanilla Cheater (about 225 calories)

½ cup unsweetened pineapple juice
½ cup skim milk
½ ripe banana
1 teaspoon vanilla extract
2 tablespoons protein powder

Cheater's Delight (about 290 calories)

½ cup papaya juice or apple juice
½ cup skim milk
1 tablespoon wheat germ
1 tablespoon of honey
½ ripe banana
2 tablespoons of protein powder

Cheater's Perfecta (about 215 calories)

½ cup skim milk
½ cup apple juice
1 whole peach (fresh)
2 tablespoons of protein powder
dash of cinnamon

Pineapple Cheater (about 240 calories)

½ cup buttermilk
½ cup unsweetened pineapple juice
3 tablespoons low-fat vanilla yogurt
2 pineapple slices
2 tablespoons protein powder

VERY IMPORTANT: You must not add any other ingredients to the preceding recipes. Also, never forget that the "Cheater Drinks" are *in place of a meal*, not *in addition* to a meal. Of course you can take vitamin pills and other supplements with your meal substitute. And make sure you drink slowly.

These four shakes, being low in calories and very nutritious, can be taken as often as once a day and help you reach your desirable weight faster with the Modified Cheater's Diet.

24

ON THE ROAD AGAIN

We must make the best of those ills which cannot be avoided. (Alexander Hamilton)

Relax. With the Cheater's Diet, eating out is a piece of cake—literally. You won't have to carry a little bag with you to restaurants, and you won't have to fight with the head waiter to order special dishes either. The diet's approach to eating out is the most versatile and practical of diets. And in no time after you start on the diet, dining out will be a cinch.

Basically, there are two ways to handle the problem of eating out.

The first and easiest approach is to plan your eating escapade so it coincides with your next cheating meal. And since you're allowed one cheating meal every four days, it will be easy to make such an arrangement. But since that cheating meal won't be taken at home and, as we know, some restaurants do have lousy service, the only restriction will be with regard to time. You will be permitted no more than an hour at the restaurant, excluding the drink you may take while you wait to order. And try to keep your meal under 1,500 calories.

The second approach to restaurants has to do with the unexpected. Let's say you just had your scheduled cheating meal for lunch at the greasy eatery next to your office. A few hours later, your workday is done and you're back home for dinner. The phone rings. It's your brother who has just come back from a four-month trip to India and he wants to dine with you in a good *American* restaurant. You can't refuse. Besides, he's paying. So you go out with him but you don't cheat on your diet. Here's how.

HOW NOT TO CHEAT AT RESTAURANTS

Here's what to do if you have to eat out frequently for business reasons. First of all, choose the restaurant *carefully*. Cheap eateries serve greasy foods. So try to select a better place to eat out. Avoid Chinese, Mexican, and Italian restaurants; their menus are too limited and their food is much too high in calories. That leaves American and French restaurants, and sea food houses. The idea behind dining out is often one of socializing as eating. So if you do as most dieters do while eating out and have only a salad, you're inviting trouble. Your friend may start to worry about your not eating enough or, worse, he or she may start teasing you about your diet. You don't need this kind of pressure.

Ideally, when you have mastered the Cheater's Diet, no one should be aware that you are on a diet. As for salad, it's mostly water and not satisfying enough for dieters. But don't get me wrong; salad is a healthy food, but you should eat something more fulfilling with it. As a rule, avoid gravy, salad oils, mayonnaise, french fries, soya sauce, and desserts. Don't add salt at all. A bit of pepper is okay. So is mustard and lemon juice as seasoning.

As for the main dish, there is plenty for you to choose from; just make sure it's done the way you order it. All good restaurants have baked potatoes (skip the butter), fish, chicken, veal, omelette, rice, and innumerable side orders of vegetables. A shrimp cocktail is delicious and can be ordered almost anywhere. Of course, you don't touch the bread and butter, which is always put on the table while you wait. Instead, you can order a glass of white wine or a light beer. But don't drink it all; apply the four-ounce rule of liquid, as with your regular meals. No one will notice how much beer you left in the bottle. In any event, stay away from hard liquors. Tomato juice is a good alternative to alcohol.

Basically, the idea of eating at restaurants is eating smaller portions than you do at home and choosing foods that are nourishing and medium or low in calories. Don't be afraid to leave a bit of everything on your plate and in your glass.

In short, there's no reason why eating out should be more difficult than eating at home, if you choose a good restaurant and keep your head. And in case you see a dish at a restaurant that you're dying to eat, tell yourself that you can always come back in a few days and eat all you want of it; that will keep you from cheating when you shouldn't.

HOW TO HANDLE PARTIES

Parties are more tricky than restaurants because you spend more time at a party. A party is *not* a place to cheat. Fortunately, there are always some veggies and crackers to munch on at gatherings. Just make sure you skip the cold meats, chips, and sauces. Hard-boiled eggs are okay. With drinks, try to stay with vegetable juice, light beer, sparkling water, or lemonade. To take your mind off the food, indulge yourself more in socializing. That's what you're there for in the first place. *Right?*

JUST LIKE MOTHER USED TO DO

If your mother invites you for dinner and it doesn't coincide with a cheating meal, use the moderate approach. Eat very small portions of everything you like (of course, only one serving); or you will have to stick to low-calorie foods and skip dessert.

EATING OUT WITH YOUR BOSS

Eating out with your boss is something special. It can make or break you, and I'm not talking about calories or pounds. The raise or promotion you've been waiting for may well depend on how you eat in front of your boss.

Never have a cheating meal when eating out with your boss. Polishing off a whole pizza before him and gulping down two or three servings of dessert can make a very bad impression on him (you know how sensitive he is). He may get the idea that you're thinking he will pay the bill or that you are lacking in self-control or both. On the other hand, if you nibble on a salad and eat nothing else, he may think you're an extremist or at least a weirdo, not so open-minded and resourceful as he had thought. Your best bet in such a situation is not to make waves; keep to the middle of the road. Do the same as if you were eating at your mother's. Order what you want and leave a bit of everything on the plate. Don't stuff yourself. Concentrate more on the conversation than on the food.

VACATION TIME

Your annual two-week vacation is coming up and you're wondering what the Cheater's Diet has in reserve for you then. Well, rejoice, because vacations should be fun. So what you have to do is this. Eat regular breakfasts and lunches that include fresh fruit and vegetables, lean meat, fish, chicken, sea food, omelette, and four ounces of unsweetened juice.

As for dinner, which is the most interesting meal on a vacation—you're allowed to cheat on it every day of your vacation. But this will be a semi-cheating meal, meaning that you will eat everything you like in moderate portions. It's the same with drinks. Variety will lend the excitement of tasting all the exotic food each country has to offer. With this cheating approach to vacations, your weight will stay the same, particularly if you walk around a lot, play tennis, and swim. But if you lie on the beach all day or cheat too much you will gain two or four pounds. However, such a small gain is well within your control; besides, it's worth the good times you've had. You'll come back home refreshed, ready to follow the Cheater's Diet with more determination than ever.

Sometimes you have to *back off* a few steps to make a bigger leap.

THE CHOICE IS YOURS

Already I hear some of you complaining that following a diet is impractical because you are always on the road or you're often in a plane. Well, I've been around a bit too and I can assure you that it's a poor excuse. The food served in most restaurants and on planes is not uncommon; *no one* can force-feed you with french fries if you don't want to. You always have a choice—even the choice of not eating at all, instead of eating junk foods. Eating is a need, but it's also a privilege. No one can prove that eating three meals a day is healthier than eating only two or one. As for running out of fuel on two meals a day, don't worry. I know many people who work very hard and who are perfectly healthy on two meals a day.

25

MONITORING YOUR PROGRESS

The penalty of success is to be bored by the attentions of people who formerly snubbed you. (M. W. Little)

The importance of this chapter may elude you at first; after all you don't have to be an Einstein to read a scale or to use a tape measure. Besides, your eyes are okay and you can see in a mirror if you're making any improvements at all. However, let me tell you that recording your progress when trying to lose weight is one of the trickiest things in the game. It can lead to despair and frustration faster than anything else I know. It can even make you quit on dieting forever.

There are many ways to monitor your progress. The most common are the scale, tape, mirror, and photos. You can use only one of them or all of them as long as you do it on a regular basis. This will let you know if you are improving or remaining at a standstill.

Now let's examine these different methods of controlling your progress.

SCALE

This instrument for weighing people has probably made more liars of people than all fishing rods put together. A lot of dieters lie consciously about their weight and a lot of others lie unconsciously because they don't know how and when to use a scale. In a 24-hour period, your body weight is about as stable as the stock market. For example, did you know that you lose over one ounce of body weight for every hour you sleep? That's one of the reasons you're always lighter in the morning. Also, did you know that after drinking two glasses of water you'll be one pound heavier? Or, that a 200-pound person can lose between four to ten pounds after two hours of vigorous exercises? Or, that there's a five-pound difference if you weigh yourself naked in the morning and then fully clothed at night?

If you want to use a scale to monitor your weight, you must have a good one to start with. That automatically excludes all the regular bathroom scales you can buy on the market; they are inaccurate—way off base. In fact, when you buy these they come with a warning paper that says they are accurate, give or take a *few* pounds. Moreover, depending on which surface you use it on (concrete, ceramic, carpet) your scale will read differently. And bathroom scales are made with springs that weaken easily after a little "family stamping."

The only scales you should use (unless you weigh more than 350 lbs.) are the medical scales (no springs) and the electronic, direct-reading scale. Of course, they are more expensive but at least you'll know the truth. If you can't afford one of them, you can use a scale at a gym or at a campus training room.

Many of you may be scale-addicts, weighing yourself each time you see one. That's no way to go. A scale is not a toy; it's an instrument of *precision*. Significant fat loss (not water) doesn't occur by the hour; it occurs by *weeks*. So when should you weigh yourself? Once a week, no more. Preferably first thing in the morning without previously eating or drinking. Empty your bladder or bowels before, if you feel the urge. Weigh yourself naked. If you can't weigh yourself in the morning or naked, the rule is to weigh yourself each week at the same hour and dressed exactly the same way each time. And always weigh yourself on the same scale.

Each weighing must serve as positive feedback for the week to come. Aim for a 2 to 4 lb. loss every week. In ten weeks that's 20 to 30 lbs., which is a lot for most dieters. Above all, remember that any weight loss, even one eighth of a pound, is a success. Be satisfied with the *smallest* loss. It adds up. Progress is in steady improvement, not in the amount involved.

If, after a weekly weighing, you find yourself at a standstill, don't be discouraged. Decrease your caloric intake significantly, not drastically. And do it on *all* the foods you eat, not just one or two. The next weighing should show a loss; if not, again decrease your consumption of all food but be sure you do it progressively. Give your body time to adapt.

TAPE

Tape measures can be as tricky as scales if you don't know how to use them. You should use a cloth or vinyl tape—no steel tapes, please. Always use the same tape. Don't let anyone measure you; measure yourself once a month (naked, it goes without saying) standing in front of a mirror. That way you won't have to make contortions to read the tape, which can lead to false measurements.

Record measurements in a book each time you take them. Always measure with tape at a right angle; avoid slanting the tape.

Here's how to measure different body parts:

Waist: At the smallest part, whether above or below the navel, body erect and stomach normally relaxed.

Chest: At the largest part right under the armpits, tape crossing shoulder blades in back and nipples in front; head up and normal breathing.

Hips: Measure where the hips are the broadest, slightly above pelvis height, and always keep your feet together.

Thigh: At the largest part of the upper thigh, feet apart, muscles relaxed.

Calf: Again, at the largest part, foot flat on the ground, muscles relaxed.

Neck: Right above the Adam's apple; keep your head straight.

Ankle: At the smallest part, feet flat on the floor.

Knee: Measure across the kneecap, muscles relaxed; straight legs are a must.

Wrist: At the smallest part, hand open, wrist as straight as possible.

Upper Arm and Forearm: Raise your arm to shoulder level, elbow bent and fist clenched, flexed hard; measure at the largest part for both muscles.

Always measure yourself in the morning before you eat or drink. This is especially important in regard to waist measurement. Even other measurements can read differently (slightly bigger) if taken in the evening.

Also, always measure both arms, legs, and calves because everyone has a difference between the right and left side. Don't worry; this asymmetry is normal.

Make sure that when you take your measurements the tape is not too loose or too tight (especially if you're very fat). The tape should fit snugly around body parts.

MIRROR

A mirror can be a useful tool in evaluating progress on the Cheater's Diet. If a scale reads 105 lbs. or a tape shows you have a 36-24-36 figure, those numbers are only indications; they are not necessarily the final proof. You can have a 36 in. hip measurement and still be plagued with cellulitis. Likewise, you can have a 36 in. bust but your breasts will lack firmness or proportion. There are too many factors involved (height, muscle tone, bone structure, muscle size, heredity) for one to assess his or her progress with numerical figures *only*. That's where a mirror comes in handy. A large, good quality mirror will give you the truth in one reflection regardless of what the scale says.

Unlike the scale or tape, the mirror should be used in early or late evening because your muscle tone is better after a day of activities and this will have an uplifting effect on your spirit. Also, when you look at yourself in the mirror, make sure you stand directly under the ceiling light. Don't stand closer than four feet from the mirror, unless you want to look bigger than you really are. As with the other methods we've discussed, there's no use checking your progress in the mirror more than once a week. And when you do, don't simply take a shy, quick look and rush off. Instead, you should be naked and you should examine your body from every angle. This should take between five and ten minutes.

As much as possible try to use the same mirror and the same lighting conditions; this way you'll be sure that the reflection you see in the glass will be true and consistent.

Remember that the scale and tape monitor the quantity of progress made; the mirror monitors its quality.

PHOTOS

Photography is another way of checking your progress while getting back in shape. It would be a good idea to have your picture taken before starting on the Cheater's Diet and then have it taken every two months or so. Have at least one taken from the front, one from the back, and one from the side. For our purposes, the photos should be in black and white and developed in matte finish. Also, use only a 35 millimeter camera with a 50 millimeter lens. Any other lens will give you a slightly distorted image. If you don't have such a camera, borrow one and ask a friend who knows something about photography to take the pictures. These photos must be taken against the same background (a dark color is best) and under the same lighting conditions for a valid evaluation of your progress.

YOUR BEST FRIENDS

When you are on a diet, your best friends can become your worst enemies, even though they are well intentioned. You should never rely on friends and family to monitor your progress in losing weight. Your friends are not experts in the field, and they are apt to be too subjective to give you honest feedback. Moreover, the way you dress has a lot to do with how heavy people think you are. Suppose one day you meet a friend you haven't seen in a long while and you are dressed in loose-fitting, long-sleeved black garments. He may say something like, "Gee, you sure have lost a lot of weight!" but, as you know very well, you are ten lbs. over your usual weight. Or, you meet the same friend two months earlier, when you were ten lbs. less than your normal weight and dressed in tight-fitting, short-sleeved white garments, and he may say, "Gee, you've gained a lot of weight lately—but that's okay, you look healthier."

Your best friend in your quest for a leaner, healthier you is the person you see in the bathroom mirror every morning. Be your own critic. You know your body better than anyone else and only you know how shapely or how slim you want to be.

The best qualities for a dieter to cultivate are *patience* and *satisfaction*. Everything worth doing is worth taking the time to do.

Part IV

Farewell Fat City

26

THE HEALTHY WAY

Some people think that doctors and nurses can put scrambled eggs back into the shell. (Dorothy Canfield Fisher)

For most people being healthy implies the absence of disease. That's one way to look at it, but I would rather think that health is the *presence* of something, namely energy, activity, and mental fitness.

After you have reached your normal body weight, not only do you have to keep it that way for the rest of your life but you also must make sure you continue in a healthy state.

It's not written anywhere that one must get sicker and sicker with old age. Certainly, we lose energy and strength as we age, but the reason we get sick more often as we age probably lies in the fact that we try to resist the evolution that takes place within our bodies. We refuse to adapt, to acknowledge that we can't put our bodies through the same stress without paying a higher price in return. Getting old in style means we have to accept the facts first, and then we have to follow our instincts as to what to eat, how much to work, and how to sleep. We must take it easy and at the same time keep active. It's more a matter of *dosage* than of restriction. We should age like some wines, getting better as we get older.

I remember a centenarian who was interviewed on television. After a brief chat, the host of the show asked him the question everybody was waiting for: "What do you think made you reach one hundred three?"

After some hesitation, the old man said, "Well, I don't know for sure, but I think it's because I started taking vitamin pills when I was ninety-five."

How old you will live has a lot to do with heredity. But whatever age you reach, the condition in which you reach it has a lot to do with your present activities. After all, there may be some truth to the saying: "Success occurs when preparation meets destiny."

Whatever your age or your present health, what you should strive for in attaining your desired weight is the *holistic* approach to health. You have to look beyond the mere mathematics of losing weight. Moral fitness, the air you breathe, the sleep you get, and the goals you set are just as important as what you eat in a day.

THE WHITE KILLERS

Anyone worth his salt knows that sodium chloride (salt) has long been associated with high blood pressure and high blood pressure is closely related to heart problems. Too much salt also can mean trouble for your kidneys. Taking these warnings from the medical field with a grain of salt might not be very wise in the long run.

Salt is a white crystaline solid, chiefly sodium chloride—40 percent sodium, 60 percent chloride—used mainly as a food seasoning and preservative. A doctor once said that salt kills what is alive and preseves what is dead. From a dieter's point of view, it's interesting to know that sodium helps retain water in the body tissues, a process you can do without. And to make matters worse, most American adults consume about 20 times their body requirements of salt. You should forever ban the utilization of the salt shaker, but even if you do, you can still consume too much salt because all processed foods contain salt or sodium. From soup to cornflakes, from soya sauce to bread, almost every food on the market contains salt. Club soda, beer, and wine contain sodium; so do frozen and canned vegetables, milk, and coke. The problem with salt is the quantity we consume. Most foods contain some quantity of natural salt. If you eat according to the Cheater's Diet, you won't have to worry about using a salt shaker anymore, except on your scheduled cheating meals.

The other white killer is sugar. In more ways than one, sugar is worse than salt. It's terrible to see a five- or six-year-old child with half his teeth rotten, but it's even more terrible when the child's parents find the situation normal.

Sugar contains only calories, and it's a robber. It robs your body of vitamin B and it can counteract the assimilation of calcium. Sugar also can induce nervousness, fatigue, skin problems, and heart diseases. To make things worse, when sugar is refined, dangerous chemicals are used to bleach the sugar to a pure, white, crystalline poison called $C_{12}H_{22}O_{11}$ or saccharose.

People are brainwashed into thinking that sugar is the supreme source of energy. Unfortunately, many uncaring or ill-advised mothers, instead of breast-feeding their newborn, prefer to give them a sweetened, canned, expensive milk substitute. And if they give the baby cow's milk, they more often than not add sugar to it, and put honey on the baby's pacifier. No wonder so many schoolchildren end up with dentures!

J. I. Rodale has said, and rightly so, that sugar is the plague of our civilization. Sugar is a dead nutriment, a drug the average American consumes in huge amounts.

SHOWERTIME

Generally speaking, blue-eyed people prefer to shower while brown- and green-eyed people would rather take a bath! Right? Well, anyway, it's a theory and I must confess that I don't have any proof. One thing I'm sure of is that, generally, people who take showers are more active and more energetic than people who take baths. What has this to do with a diet book? A lot indeed. Beyond the superior cleaning aspect of showers is the fact that baths are emollients and showers are energizers.

For one thing a bath—particularly a long and hot one—softens your muscles and skin, and by overrelaxing yourself, you *weaken* your willpower. So, to reinforce your successful dieter's profile and to make your approach to the Cheater's Diet more holistic, avoid taking baths on a regular basis. When you do take one, make it short and in lukewarm water. Moreover, a hot bath is the last thing you should indulge in if you are plagued with varicose veins; it would only aggravate your condition.

On the other hand, showers are usually shorter than baths, and they should be taken with lukewarm water. Also, when you shower, oxygen from the running water is liberated. That's one of the reasons you feel so energetic after a shower. As a bonus, showers give you the added benefit of a light massage, which is good for your skin and muscle tone. So don't lie anymore; stand up to shower power!

TAKE IT EASY

One criterion for success in dieting, or in any other endeavor for that matter, is control over outward and inward pressure in our lives. Inward pressure is particularly difficult to master because it's directly related to emotions. Suppose you've just started to diet and your spouse asks for a divorce or you lose your job. This kind of inward pressure can quickly ruin your diet plans. But sometimes that kind of emotional upset can have the opposite effect, and you end up the winner because of the challenge and stimulation provided by such situations. The way we handle inward pressure is rather personal and there's no sure-fire cure, except perhaps time and determination to get over your problem.

Outward pressure is more subtle but is a most important factor in your failure to diet successfully or to stay at your normal weight once you have reached it. For outward pressure has to do with your everyday living, your life-style.

Who says you have to rush to work every morning? Get up early. Take it easy. Take control over simple things like that. Why be a slave to the phone each time it rings? If you don't feel like answering, don't. Just try once to deliberately let it ring until it stops. You'll be surprised at the overpowering feeling of control you'll get.

Don't let your noisy kids make a nervous wreck out of you. And don't get upset when you're caught in a traffic jam. There's nothing you can do about it anyway.

Most people don't think; they act like robots, not because they are not intelligent but because they are programmed (mainly by publicity) to act that way. But people are not machines, and all this stress and conditioned behavior builds up outward pressure, resulting in loss of self-control. This is bad for anyone, particularly someone who is trying to lose weight. You cannot separate the mind from the body—you are what *you think*.

27

THE SECOND MOST IMPORTANT CHAPTER

Energy: that's what life is all about. (Vince Gironda)

If it's true that energy is what life is all about, it also must be true that movement is what energy is all about. Movement produces or transmits motion, thus creating energy. And ever since the dawn of time, our cultural inheritance has been affected by movement. We find movement everywhere: in labor, music, prose, arts. And what else but movement created the Egyptian pyramids and other such wonders?

Would you believe that Greek philosophers like Plato and Aristotle claimed that walking created the ideal condition for thinking?

Einstein's theory of relativity was formulated through a study of movement in space and time. So we can see that anything of value, any great discovery or achievement in this world, has been the result of movement and energy (directly and indirectly)—not of dozing off in a chair all day long.

Now before you start thinking that I am a case for the men in the white coats because of my delirious prose (I know this book is about dieting, but dieting is about losing weight and in losing weight *everything* matters), let's get to the point of this chapter—the physical aspect of reducing.

The question is, what part does exercise play in the Cheater's Diet? Simply put, it's the prerequisite of success. But not for the reasons you may think. Certainly, exercise burns up calories and it's a welcome bonus; however, it's easier to put on calories than it is to get rid of them. Anyone in his right mind would agree it's easier to eat two servings of hot apple pie than it is to ride a stationary bike for two hours. Yet eating the pie, besides your regular meals, add up to 800 extra calories and biking for two hours burns about 800 calories. Are you ready to put in two hours of exercise for every five-minute eating binge? Probably not and neither am I.

So it must be clear by now that you can exercise vigorously for hours every day and still be fat because it's easier to stock calories than it is to use them up and because most fat people are born with rather slow metabolism.

Trying to diet without exercising is like trying to make love without taking off your clothes first! I know it can be done, but both are harder and more frustrating. So why trek through the woods like a savage when you can cruise on the freeway like a civilized person?

If you ever had a limb in a cast for weeks or months, you have witnessed the damage immobility causes to a body part. It reduces the size and the tone of the supporting muscles, weakens bones and ligaments, and impairs the coordination and vitality of the part immobilized. This will make you realize the truth behind the following biological statement: The function creates the organ. It's a case of using it or losing it. However, the real benefits of exercise for a dieter are of a *psychological* nature. Here's why. Simply put, to lose weight you have to eat a lot less. But eating a lot less long enough to lose weight is the tricky part.

Fortunately, the fundamental principle of the Cheater's Diet, allowing you to cheat on one meal every four days, comes to the rescue by preventing a buildup of frustration. But what about the more subtle, every-day cheating in the form of excuses? This is where exercise enters the picture. Any person who has exercised long enough (at least three times a week over a three-month period) can vouch that it's easy to follow a diet when you regularly engage in physical activity. When these same people take a prolonged holiday from such activities, they start eating junk foods regularly and are unable to resist temptation, no matter how hard they try. Why exercise makes a tremendous difference between successful dieting and unsuccessful dieting is still not fully understood. However, one thing is sure, it *works*. The way I see it, exercise acts unconsciously on the mind of the dieter as self-hypnosis. Every repetition, every movement, every effort made in the gym is a suggestion sent to the brain. This phenomenon strengthens willpower like nothing else can.

Another reason to explain the determination imparted to dieters who exercise might be found in the well-known "high" experienced after 30 minutes to one hour of doing vigorous activities. Perhaps reaching that stage of euphoria lessens the need for another sensual pleasure—eating.

Moreover, exercise is a great relaxer. A person who is relaxed has more control over his actions and thus is not likely to yield to impulsive eating.

Exercise alone won't do much to help you lose weight, but coupled with the cheating method explained earlier, it is indeed *half* the battle.

BREATHING AND LONELINESS

The first and foremost nutriment is air. Sixty days without food can kill you and so can a week without water. Yet if you stop breathing for only a few minutes you can make an undertaker somewhere very happy.

From your first breath till your last, what keeps you alive is the air that reaches your lungs; unless that air is clean, you shorten your stay in this world. Biologists tell us that people, like some animals, are genetically programmed to live seven times the period it takes them to reach maturity. Thus if we assume a man or woman reaches maturity at twenty (some experts say it's more like twenty-five) and multiply by seven we reach the awesome age-figure of 140. On the other hand, some people who smoke two packs of cigarettes a day die of heart attack or cancer in their early fifties.

Breathing is never so important as when you exercise. Your body is then submitted to additional stress and requires more oxygen to clean your blood faster, thus permitting you to carry on with a greater work load. Yet one of the greatest myths in regard to exercise is inhaling and exhaling air. Many people think that if you exhale during a specific exercise when you should be inhaling (or vice versa), you negate the benefits of the exercise. Nothing is farther from the truth. Respiration is the most natural thing your body can do. It will let you know when it needs more air. So don't worry. The only way you can go wrong is when you hold your breath while exerting yourself. If you do that you'll feel dizzy and you can even pass out. So the first rule while exercising is to breathe freely—never *hold* your breath.

The second rule is to breathe deeply. When you go to gyms and spas, you see some people who are too shy to breathe deeply, as if they were afraid of taking in all the air in the room. Of course you don't have to puff like a sumo wrestler but you should make a conscious effort to breathe more deeply than you normally do.

The third and last rule applies to certain body building exercises such as sit-ups, pull-overs, and lateral flies. You should exhale when you fold your body, as in a sit-up and inhale when you stretch your body, as in a straight arm pull-over. Breathing this way makes such exercises easier to do.

Remember, don't worry about when to inhale and when to exhale. Just make sure you breathe freely and deeply while exercising.

Following a diet and exercising have two things in common. Both are solitary but rewarding experiences. That is, they should be. You should not depend on someone else to start on a diet or to join a gym. Fitness is something you achieve alone. Yet you don't have to be antisocial. If you begin to diet or exercise with someone else, you will feel a terrible let-down if a few weeks later, he or she quits. That doesn't mean you can't start on the Cheater's Diet with your spouse or join a gym with your girlfriend, but don't compromise in any way just to please others and don't expect them to stay by your side for long. Don't let them control any part of your diet or exercise program. Build up your own self-motivation. Be a leader, not a follower. If you wait for someone to help you start dieting or exercising you are on the road to failure.

Do it alone and you will reach your goal faster.

EXERCISES AND PSEUDO-EXERCISES

The word exercise has more than one definition. The one we will deal with here is the following: an activity that requires physical or mental exertion, especially when performed to develop or maintain fitness. After a careful study of this definition, we can conclude that there is real exercise and pseudo-exercise (bowling, walking, golf, snowmobile, riding, etc.). Don't get me wrong; I have nothing against pseudo-exercise, as long as you do real exercise as well. Take bowling, for example. It's not a real exercise; it's a game, that's all. But all games aren't pseudo-exercises. Racquetball is a game but it requires physical exertion. And I agree with you that golf requires a good swing but the lapse of time between each stroke is too long and the idea behind golf is not to develop fitness but to go through the course averaging as few shots as possible.

Walking is probably the biggest pseudo-exercise of them all. Many lazy people will boast about the advantages of walking because they think the only alternative to it is running. To most of us, walking is second nature. We've been walking for years, so our bodies have adjusted economically to this minor form of activity. Walking can do no more than take you from point A to point B, unless you do it at a fast pace and all day long, like a postman does. Have you ever seen an obese postman? Neither have I.

Yet walking fast all day long will not make you fat-free, if you consume calories in excess of your daily needs. Then why is the postman not obese? It's more a question of temperament than of calories burned up in a day. People who apply as postmen are generally of the nervous-active type with fast or medium metabolisms. They choose this job because they like moving fast, and they like moving fast because of their temperament. On the other hand, the last thing a lympatic-type individual wants to do is deliver mail with great speed all day long.

From a dieter's point of view, a good exercise should increase your blood circulation, your respiration rhythm, and your heartbeat. Moreover, you should be able to increase the intensity of the exercise as you become more efficient at it. In short, you should exert yourself without reaching exhaustion.

The best exercises to do (in no specific order) are the following:

swimming, biking, running, jogging, skipping rope, body building, basketball, handball, and tennis. This list is not complete but it gives you an idea of the kinds of exercise you should indulge in if you want to resist temptation and burn up extra calories.

Of course if, for any medical reason, you can't do these activities, don't fret about it. Try to develop your willpower by some form of suggestive meditation. Or, if the idea of going to the pool or jogging around the block embarrasses you, join a gym. No one will laugh at you there. Like you, they want to better themselves. They will understand how you feel and they'll try to help you.

There's always the alternative of waiting until you have shed some of your fat before getting involved in a particular activity. But don't wait too long. As soon as you feel ready, get a physical checkup and go ahead with your new life.

HOW MUCH IS ENOUGH?

Any exercise or activity performed less than *three times a week* will not produce the desired results. As to the duration of a session, anything under one hour is of little value, except for jogging and running. Look at it this way. It takes about 15 minutes to warm up the body properly, so if you do a one-hour session, you are actually getting 45 minutes of result-producing exercise. Beware of fraudulent publicity that claims you can attain fitness by using an expensive gimmick five or ten minutes a day. Even some physical educators who have nothing to sell—nothing except an idea—may tell you less than the truth. Why? They don't want to turn people off by telling them that to attain fitness, three or four sessions of one hour to one-and-a-half hours are required weekly.

When you tell people it takes four to six hours a week of exercising to be in shape, they hit the roof. Where would they find those precious hours? Yet, curiously, those same people sit in front of the tube for 20 to 30 hours a week!

For most dieters, a few hours of exercising each week is the wisest move they can make toward a slim and sexy body.

EXTRA BONANZA

In addition to helping you lose weight, exercise can reduce your heartbeat. Generally, heartbeat ranges between 60 to 90 pulsations a minute; for most people, the average is 72 beats. Among obese people, over 100 beats a minute is not uncommon. So the higher your pulse, the more unfit you are, and the lower it is, the more fit you are likely to be. When your heart works more economically, it lasts longer, just as a car motor running regularly at 50 miles an hour will outlast one that is continually run at top speed.

When you take your pulse make sure you are in a resting state. The wrist or the neck is the best place to take your pulse. Count the beats for 15 seconds, then multiply that amount by four. That gives you your pulse for a minute. My pulse rate has been as high as 80 after a prolonged layoff from exercise and as low as 48 when in contest-shape. Marathon runners average between 28 and 36 beats a minute.

Hypertension is another villain that exercise can help ward off. By reducing your weight, you can reduce blood pressure and lessen the chance of developing heart trouble. And that's a solace in view of the fact that heart attack is the nation's number-one killer.

Depression, anxiety—any kind of emotional stress—can be greatly relieved through vigorous exercise. People who get physical on a regular basis rarely wind up on the analyst's couch. In the event of emotional distress, such as a divorce or the death of a loved one, exercise can be of great help in coping. When situations like that arise, people who are not physically active run a greater chance of getting involved with drugs or booze. Emotional problems cause mental wounds that can be healed in the long run; by exercising, keeping the mind occupied, and helping the stressed body to relax, you can speed up the process of psychic healing.

Last but not least, there's a big "plastic" advantage to exercising while on a diet, especially if you're many pounds overweight. Many obese people find their ideal body weight only to end up with another problem: the loose-skin "garment." And it's not merely a matter of losing fat too fast or of being over 30. The skin didn't spring back on the new body mainly because no exercise was done to coax it into snapping back. Exercise, by toning muscles and by feeding skin with ample amounts of fresh blood, takes care of this unsightly problem of loose skin after reducing. But there's only one kind of exercise that will resolve the problem of loose skin perfectly and it's body building. Biking won't make the sagging skin on your chest tighter. Jogging won't do a thing for the flabby skin on the back of your arms, and tennis won't improve your flaccid stomach. Only *specific exercises* for specific body parts will assure the resilience of your skin.

If you have a lot of weight to lose or want to make sure you don't end up with loose skin, the best thing to do is to join a gym. But be sure to start your exercises as soon as you begin on the Cheater's Diet, for if you wait until your skin is loose, it might be next-to-impossible to get it tight again.

Also, choose a gym where you can work on apparatus and with barbells and dumbbells—not just free-hand exercises.

The best example of someone who shed a lot of weight and kept perfectly tight skin is Bruce Randall. At a body weight of 401 lbs., Bruce started dieting but kept on training with weights. Thirty-two weeks later, he weighed only 183 lbs., a reduction of 218 lbs. and no flabby skin. Bruce continued to train and went on to win the Mr. Universe Contest in London. Years later, I met him in Montreal where he was giving a fitness seminar in a downtown mall, and his skin was still beautifully tight on his herculean body.

Will it to be possible, and you can do it.

IMPROVING YOUR SELF-IMAGE

Next to losing weight, exercise is the best thing you can do to improve your self-image. Surprisingly enough, most people who join a gym are reluctant to admit that they wish to alter the shape of their body. Most of them talk about the health aspects of training, implying that they aren't body-conscious. Yet, if people went to gyms only to benefit their health, *all* gyms in America would have closed their doors a long time ago. Ninety-five percent of the people who reduce their body weight do it primarily because they are self-conscious. Sure, they don't mind being healthy but for most of them it's more or less a pleasant side effect.

Who doesn't look at himself in a mirror at least once a day? We are a nation of body-conscious people and there's nothing wrong with that; it is a part of our evolution, of having one of the highest standards of living in the civilized world. And we are brainwashed by T.V., newspapers, magazines, and radio to want to look good all the time. But such artificial standards may not be desirable. Women with silicone breasts, wigs, and super-white painted teeth are not exactly what we can call natural women. And all those artificial means will prove a big letdown when they fade. A well-developed, fit, and strong body obtained through a vigorous exercise program, along with the Cheater's Diet, will bring you unexpected rewards, well above the mere fact of having attained your desired body weight. Why play with only half a deck of cards? A serious, regular exercise program is indeed the *second most important move* you can make to reach your goal. So put a sweatband on your head, if you like, but make sure you get physical.

28

FOOD FOR THOUGHT

Learning without thought is labor lost. (Confucius)

Your body is everything you have. The only freedom a healthy person has in this world is the freedom of thought. The road to health must be a big party: You do the exercises you like, you take the supplements you like, you thrive on the Cheater's Diet, and above all, you keep company with friends who share your philosophy of life.

The world belongs to the adventurers and the dreamers.
The only drama in life is to get out of it.

If your gums bleed, you should eat more vitamin C foods. Kiwi fruits are a much better source of vitamin C than oranges. Besides, oranges are immersed in a harmful chemical (biphenyl) so they won't ripen too fast.

Believe it or not, coffee, tea, chocolate, white sugar, and tobacco are drugs. A drug is an addictive substance and, by extension, a poison. There's even a newsletter for chocolate addicts around the world that is published in the United States.

Some experts in nutrition claim that vitamin B-15 is the miracle of the century. Others say it doesn't even exist.

The average North American takes about *ten pounds* of pure chemicals a year mainly through food consumption. I strongly believe that the synergetic interaction of all those chemicals is the main cause of cancer.

Frying foods doubles their calorie content. Example: Half a chicken breast steam cooked without its skin yields 117 calories while the same piece, fried with skin, amounts to 241 calories.

A small apple yields 64 calories as well as some complex carbohydrates (needed for energy). Besides, it's a better breath-freshner than any mouthwash on the market (kills more bacteria). An apple a day keeps your lover on the way.

One soft drink taken every night before going to bed will make you ten pounds heavier in a year, if it's in excess of your calorie requirements.

The worse thing you can put into your body on a daily basis is that stuff called "orange juice," which is made by adding crystal powder to water. Margarine is not too far behind; it can be made with just about anything.

Women, especially after pregnancy, as well as those who have large breasts, often end up with unsightly stretch marks on their skin. These are usually located on the stomach or on the upper chest. With men, this condition is found mostly among body builders, occurring in the shoulder-chest connection near the armpit. In both men and women, this condition is caused by a breakdown of capillaries submitted to too much stretching. If you want to get rid of stretch marks, try this formula for three months: Take (daily) 10,000 I.U. of vitamin A, three kelp tablets, and be sure to eat enough vitamin C foods, such as tomatoes, cantaloupe, broccoli, kiwi (the fruit, not the bird), and potatoes. Also, rub some vitamin E oil on your stretch marks once a day, especially before you exercise—it will not speed up the healing process but it can prevent further damage to the skin.

Ice cream contains 20 percent sugar, a lot of fat, and many other ingredients you wouldn't believe.

A study on coffee showed that the equivalent of four cups produced birth defects in rats when taken daily. Tea is even worse, containing more than twice as many toxins as coffee. Adding insult to injury, tea stains your teeth and gives you bad breath.

Domestic animals (horses, cows, dogs) are better fed than the average American. They get oatmeal, wheat, black-strap molasses, and bran, while we poor humans have residual white flour and white sugar.

The mind is the jailer of the body; it can set you free in time or keep you in for life.

Oil (cooking or salad) is the most concentrated source of calories you can put into your body; one pound yields 4,013 calories. Margarine follows with 3,275 calories and butter is not far behind with 3,250 a pound. Think about that the next time you get the "greasies" and want to reach for an o-i-l-y dish.

Recent medical reports indicate that low-fat diets can greatly reduce the symptoms of arthritis. The Cheater's Diet is essentially low in fat.

If you are always tired the best thing you can do to ward off fatigue, besides exercising, is to take raw wheat germ and desiccated liver tablets every day. Both are good sources of B vitamins, and desiccated liver (Argentinian liver is best) has a fatigue-fighter pigment protein (P-450). Also, a 45-minute nap after coming home from work (more than that has been proven useless in experiments) can increase your energy for the rest of the day by 25 percent.

Note: Argentinian liver, desiccated and defatted, is especially useful to help prevent anemia because it's rich in vitamin B-12 and iron. As we all know, anemia is a major cause of fatigue.

Some experts in nutrition believe that oatmeal (for its fiber content) and apples (for its pectin) when eaten regularly can prevent cholesterol buildup on arterial walls.

Forks kill more people than switch-blade knives.

Exercise and get smarter. A study in an American university on a group of middle-aged men indicated that after a program of vigorous exercises (an hour and a half, three times a week) the men showed greater efficiency of the brain's left hemisphere. They showed improvement in problem-solving tests, unlike those in the controlled group who did not exercise. The theory behind this improvement is that exercising increases the level of glucose in the blood, the brain thrives on glucose for nourishment.

29

FORTY-SIX DIETER'S HELPERS

The essence of knowledge is, having it, to apply it; not having it, to confess your ignorance. (Confucius)

The following is a smorgasborg of tips, tricks and hints that can make dieting easier for you. Some of them are directly related to dieting and some are not; however, don't underestimate the power of these psychological tricks. Remember: Dieting is easy—but only when you've got the proper tools to work with and know how to use them adequately.

1. This first hint is perhaps the daddy of them all. It can help you save between 15 to 30 percent on your grocery bill. Here it is: Always do your grocery shopping about half an hour after a high-protein meal and when stores are less crowded.

Eating less, that's what losing weight is all about. It's *easier* to avoid temptation by having the right food in your fridge than trying to resist it. So, out of sight, out of mind. A high-protein meal will raise your blood-sugar; you will feel fulfilled (with less calories) and in perfect control. Then you'll be able to choose only the foods you really want to buy.

2. Always believe that you will succeed. Always "see" yourself at your ideal weight. Maybe, in the long run, you are what you eat, but more important, you are *what you think you are*.

3. If you are a woman, go to the hairdresser more often.

4. If you are a man, always shave first thing in the morning—even on your days off.

5. Whenever you feel like cheating and you shouldn't, try to draw your attention away from food: go out to the library, go see an exposition or just take a walk. If, for whatever reason, you can't go out, take a few glasses of cool water and call a friend. You can also take a shower or, best of all, do some exercises for the stomach.

6. Never bet with friends, family members, or co-workers that you can lose X amount of weight in a certain period of time; it's the worst thing you can do. Deadlines mean pressure, which is the last thing you need to succeed.

7. Remember that you must combine diet and exercise for best results. The most enjoyable and efficient program of exercise a dieter can do is: 45 minutes of body building, followed by 20 minutes of stationary bike. To finish the session, take a 20-minute swim. Do this four or five times a week for best results.

8. Develop your willpower by daily acts that require effort on your part; for example, waiting half an hour before opening your mail (not the bills, that's easy).

9. Dress to create an illusion of slimness: vertical stripes or designs, darker colors, lighter garment tissues (heavy corduroy makes you look extra fat) and so forth. It will strengthen your determination and it'll keep you working on your body.

10. Do not let the amount of weight you have to lose discourage you. Think in terms of short-range goals; for example, 10 to 15 pounds in a month. Don't rush the process of shedding weight. By not rushing the process, there will be less stress on your system, and you will have a chance to adapt to your newly found body.

11. Don't sleep too much. When you wake up, don't stay in bed for another hour. Instead, get up and do something.

12. Use self-hypnosis to focus your mental power on your goals of losing weight. Before falling asleep at night and whenever you think about it, repeat mentally, and many times, the following suggestion: I will reach the body weight I want with the Cheater's Diet.

13. Get yourself into some kind of physical sports or activities that involve the biggest muscle group of the body, the thighs. For example: squatting exercises, racquetball, skipping rope, running. This way you'll burn up more calories and your cardiovascular system will greatly benefit too.

14. Lower back pain can affect your spirit and your spirit can affect your diet to a great extent. To prevent or relieve lower back problems, hang from a chinning bar (loosely) for up to a minute, twice a day or more.

15. Never eat when you are sick. Do as animals do; take a nap. The energy that would have been used to digest food is used instead to fight your illness.

16. About once a week, skip a meal, preferably lunch or dinner. But, and here lies the secret, never forget to use this spare time to do half an hour to one hour of vigorous exercise (your choice). You won't believe how easy it is to skip a meal without feeling hungry. (The more vigorous the exercise, the easier it will be.) And when you skip a meal, don't plan it; do it on the spur of the moment when you really feel like doing it.

17. Don't fall into an eating rut. Use your imagination to create your own favorite low-calorie natural recipes. (Mine is skinless chicken breasts with a side dish of garlic brown rice, seasoned with fresh lime juice. Delicious!)

18. Any kind of smoking is bad for you as a dieter. It *weakens* your will and *robs* you of precious energy that could otherwise be used to reach your ideal body weight. Smoking also deadens your sense of taste by clogging your taste buds with tar and other poisons. No wonder smokers have to put so much salt on their foods!

19. Develop the habit of leaving a little bit of everything on your plate and a few sips in your cup or glass. In two weeks you will feel and see the difference—that is, if you take a small serving of food or drink to begin with. Otherwise you'll only be fooling yourself.

20. Don't stay idle on your days off. You can't expect to lose weight if you spend all your free time on the couch. Be a doer, not a dozer.

21. If you are craving sugar all the time, you probably need more protein. Decrease your carbohydrates (fruits, bread) and increase your protein intake with such items as chicken (without skin), turkey, veal, lamb, lean fish, eggs, mozzarella cheese, and plain yogurt. Try a dash of cinnamon, or a teaspoonful of honey and a few drops of vanilla extract to flavor yogurt. Really peachy!

22. When you weigh yourself once a week and have lost some body weight (even as little as one-eighth of a pound), then and *only then*, reward yourself. Buy yourself some nice clothing, a good book, or something else you want.

23. Take a few minutes before you fall asleep each night to plan your next day. Visualize how much control you will have over your food and how much closer to your goal you will be.

24. If you feel like munching all the time in the first few weeks on the Cheater's Diet, munch on celery or carrots. You can't go wrong because you burn up about as many calories in chewing than the stick contains.

25. Keep a stationary bicycle in your living room. Then, when you are watching your favorite TV program, jump on your bike during the commercial break and give it a smooth ride until the show resumes. Because there are so many commercials today, you could easily average more than an hour of exercise in a week.

26. Don't be a fanatic about your diet. Don't bore your friends with diet considerations—especially if they are non-dieters. The negative pressure you could then build up around you is a no-no. You don't need that. Preach by the example you set; you won't lose friends and you will gain the respect of everyone.

27. If your enthusiasm for dieting is dwindling and you are on the verge of giving up, go see a body building contest. It's the best panacea I know of. Nothing like the spectacle of those almost-perfect bodies can reinforce your will to diet. Even if you are not a body building fan you will be inspired by the unyielding dedication of those men and women (who were once like you).

28. Keep your life in order. Try to resolve your conflict (marital, familial, sexual, or job-related) that messes up your life. Stressful situations can play havoc with your diet.

29. Go out every day to get a little sunshine and a lot of fresh air. Walk slowly and do some deep breathing to rid your body of its impurities. Don't forget that air is the first and foremost nutrient.

30. Never eat a food you don't like. You don't have to. Each food has a substitute that will do as good a job to feed your body properly. Likewise for exercise—don't swim if what you like is dancing, don't jog if you would rather be pumping iron, and so on.

31. If you are living with people who don't have a weight problem and the fridge is always full of goodies, put a photo (you know, the one you hate) of yourself on the fridge door at eye level. That might just do it for you.

32. Learn all you can about your body's internal mechanisms and about nutrition. Be proud to know how your body works and what makes it run efficiently.

33. Don't be afraid to sweat. Indulge in as many physical activities (yes, including that one) as you can. Get moving—you will burn up calories and you will keep your mind occupied.

34. Create your own weight reducing motto (keep it short). Write it down and put it where you can see it every day. Suggestion: *Get slim while you can.*

35. Always dress as if you were going out. Choose joyful, tasteful, youthful designs; it will reinforce your self-image and your will to diet.

36. The best thing you can do after a meal is relax. Don't do anything strenuous, this would only upset your digestion—the stomach needs blood to digest food. Good digestion means good assimilation and good assimilation means more energy from the nutrients you eat. You won't be hungry so soon after a meal if you make a habit of relaxing for ten to fifteen minutes after each meal.

37. Try to hang around with friends who respect your concern for health and who encourage you to keep on dieting. Don't be misled by the "we-like-you-as-you-are" statement.

38. Whenever you can, do some stomach exercises (bent-legs sit-up, bent legs up) before going to bed. Do them very slowly. Five to ten minutes is enough. You will sleep better and will have used up some calories in the process. Remember—it's what you do every day that makes the difference.

39. Don't make excuses for cheating on your diet when you shouldn't. If one excuse is good, you will likely use it again. Then success will slip away from you. If you don't succeed people won't ask you why, but if you win, you can be sure they will ask you how you did it.

40. Some nights you will come home so hungry you can eat a horse. Don't! Instead, eat some fruits (banana, kiwi, grapes, apple). Then prepare your main dish. Take your time. Fruit sugar is quickly absorbed by the body and this will curb your hunger for the meal to come.

41. Be kind to yourself. Show respect for your body—get a medical checkup at least once a year (even if you feel healthy, it's better to be safe than sorry) and get your teeth cleaned by a dentist every six months or so. In short, treat your body for what it is: *your most precious possession*.

42. Read autobiographies of people who fought their way to the top. You'll be inspired and nothing will seem too big to be accomplished in the future.

43. Keep your goal in mind all the time but don't be obsessed by your diet to the point of being self-centered. Take an active part in some charitable cause or join a nonprofit social club.

44. Do you feel lifeless and bloated all the time due to constipation? Here's what to do: avoid white bread, white flour products, and hard cheese. Drink enough water (especially on arising), eat more fresh fruit and vegetables, and take one tablespoonful of bran (no more) daily in half a glass of water, juice, or yogurt. Last but not least, do two series of 20 bent-legs sit-ups each night before going to bed. In a few weeks you'll feel light and lively again.

45. If you live alone get yourself a pet (dog, cat, parrot). You'll feel less lonely, you'll have someone to care for, and to talk to, and you'll be kept busy and as happy as a kid. Moreover, if you buy a dog, he'll be begging for his walk everyday and that's good for you too.

46. At this point in the book there may still be some unanswered questions in your mind pertaining to diet, exercise, or fitness in general. If so, you can write to me for personal advice. Send me a one-page letter stating your age, sex, occupation, nationality, weight, height, measurements, plus a *specific* description of your problem. Also a recent photo would help.

Include a self-addressed stamped envelope and a twenty-dollar money order. I will be glad to help you.

        Send to: Daniel Tremblay
                 1641 Alcide
                 Brossard, Qué
                 Canada
                 J4W IZ9

30

FOOD SUPPLEMENTS

In everything the middle road is the best; all things in excess bring trouble to men. (Plautus)

Any book on diets without a chapter on food supplements would be either incomplete or not serious. The market for food supplements is growing at a prodigious rate, particularly in North America where suplements are a multimillion-dollar business.

Lately, along with the spectacular fitness craze, supplements have been invading our visual environment. Besides the health food store, you can now find so-called "natural" products everywhere: drugstores, grocery stores, sport shops, gyms, spas, etc. I bet a friend of yours is even selling them in his basement.

We can conclude, therefore, that many people are still searching for the mythical fountain of youth or some kind of elixir that would rid them of disease and guarantee them a longer stay on the good old planet earth.

The controversy about supplements rages on. Experts in the field have yet to reach accord on the subject. In regard to health products, you usually get two kinds of reactions from people: a smile (incredulous) or a serious look. I, for one, believe in supplements—having personally experimented with about all the market has to offer. But I do have reservations about supplements.

The question that may be on your mind is: "Is it necessary that I take food supplements in conjunction with the Cheater's Diet to achieve success?"

The answer is no—absolutely not. You don't have to; it's optional. To show you what I mean by *optional,* suppose you have been gazing at the car of your dreams in the showroom for half an hour. Now you're sitting in the office with the salesman. The car you want to buy is a mid-size beauty-of-the-year by the famous brand X auto maker. The price is right but you don't like the color. So you decide to order one with the features you like. Then comes a few questions. The salesman asks you if you want the standard four-cylinder motor or the optional six-cylinder—which costs an extra $300.

Now you have a tough decision to make. Sure, a four-cylinder would be more economical and you would always get from point A to point B without much trouble, you think to yourself. But then you begin to wonder. Maybe when you want to pull your boat this summer it will be a real drag; and maybe when you have to pass another car on the highway you will mutter some naughty words to yourself and maybe . . . Well, you get the picture.

So you have to decide whether the few hundred bucks you'll save each year in gas is worth the hassle. Likewise, you have to decide whether a few hundred dollars spent each year on supplements is worth the health benefits.

I have always strived to increase my energy potential in a healthy way. We've only got one life to live and what's a few hundred dollars a year anyway. Most people who smoke spend about twice as much and those who drink regularly easily spend more than four times this amount annually. So *you* decide; it's your move. But first we'll take a closer look at supplements.

WHAT ARE THEY?

Supplements are either completely concentrated foods or concentrated extracts of food. In either case, they are nutrients and nutriments, put on the market to supply our diet with adequate amounts of vitamins, minerals, enzymes, and proteins. Most regular foods are so processed with chemicals of all kinds (additives, preservatives, colorants, flavoring) that what is left on the shelf at the supermarket hardly does anything to keep you alive and healthy. Certainly I wouldn't qualify supplements as super foods. They are only the second best thing to truly natural food; but since not many people grow their own fruit anymore and hardly anyone keeps beef and chicken in the backyard to supply meat and eggs, food supplements do have their place in your home today. Moreover, if you add to this, air pollution, the stress of big-city life, smoking, drinking and depletion of the soil caused by industrial farming, you can see that our bodies will welcome the extra help that supplements bring.

THE FEAR-OF-THE-PILL SYNDROME

Picture this: A young man in his early twenties is sitting alone in a restaurant. He has just finished his lunch. Two women sitting nearby are watching him from time to time, for the guy looks tall and he's good looking.

Suddenly the young man takes a little bag out of his pocket and starts to pop pills of different colors, sizes, and shapes. He washes all this down with a glass of water and looks rather relieved and satisfied.

The women are shocked. It happened right before their eyes in broad daylight. "The guy must be very ill to take all that medication," says one of the women. "I'm sure he's a dopehead," says the other woman.

Curiosity getting the best of them, the two women get up, and ask the young man why he took so many pills. He answers that they were only food supplements: vitamins, minerals, proteins, etc.

"Didn't I tell you," says one of the women. "He's not a dopey. They were just vitamin pills."

"I don't care what he said or what you think," says the other woman, vexed. "Pills are pills, that's all—let's get out of here!"

This scenario shows you the narrow-mindedness of some people. A pill is not only a pill. It can be a tablet, a capsule, a pellet—it could be anything. One thing is sure, however; for most people anything that is *shaped* like a pill is bad. People lack discernment because they aren't well informed; they equate vitamin pills with medication. The former is a nutriment and the latter is a drug. You have to look beyond appearance, beyond the shape or package in which things come.

Take a wheat germ capsule, for example. This is a capsule made of gelatin (protein from animal sources) containing a little oil obtained by pressing large amounts of raw, 100 percent whole wheat. It is totally different from a medication pill (drug), which is made in laboratories with 100 percent pure chemicals.

The same thing is true of a desiccated liver tablet. Liver tablets are made with liver from which the water and fat have been removed. What remains is a product that is more powerful (concentrated) than the original source. Unlike regular liver, liver tablets are eaten raw. This way nutrients are not destroyed by heat but are concentrated to make a better food product.

Remember that supplements and regular foods do have something in common. You can find good supplements and bad supplements in a health food store, just as you can find bad foods and good foods at the supermarket.

Each time you eat or drink something, you take a risk; it could be a long-term risk or a short-term one. Only time will tell.

So be aware, ask questions and, above all, read labels. In short, keep yourself well informed. There's no excuse not to be.

MEGADOSE: A NO-NO

Among people who are convinced of the value of food supplements, the biggest controversy is probably related to dosage. On one side, you have those who believe that supplements should be taken as indicated on the manufacturer's label, or according to the F.D.A. recommendations (which are usually lower). On the other side, you have those who swear by huge dosages in the belief that such dosages can cure everything from soft nails to cancer.

What is a megadose?

In terms of food supplements, a megadose is ten times the minimum daily intake recommended by the Food and Drug Administration for a particular vitamin.

For example, the F.D.A. has established the minimum daily requirement for vitamin C at 60 milligrams; we multiply by ten and find that 600 mg of C is the megadose. Likewise, if we take vitamin E (potency is calculated in International Units instead of milligrams) we can say that a megadose starts at 300 I.U.s—the M.D.R. for vitamin E being 30 I.U.s.

Now that you have an idea of what a megadose of supplements is, let's see why megadoses are a no-no.

To begin with, what are the functions of vitamins in the human body? Vitamins are complex organic substances found in plants and animal tissues. They are essential in small amounts for the control of metabolic processes. Compared to fat, protein and carbohydrates, the proportion of vitamins required by the body is *minute*. There is a good reason for this. Although vitamins are essential to the development of your body, their energetic and "block building" properties are almost nil. Unlike fat, vitamins can't give you a lot of calories; unlike protein, they don't build your muscles; and unlike carbohydrates, they don't give you energy.

So what's all the fuss about? Why does everyone seem ready to jump on the megadose bandwagon? Because most people think that if one capsule of vitamin is good for them, two capsules will be twice as good. But it doesn't work that way. You have to draw a line somewhere. If you don't, your body will.

There are two groups of vitamins: fat-soluble (A, D, E, K) and water-soluble (B, C, Folic acid, Biotin, Pantothenic acid, Chlorine, Inositol, PABA).

The fat-soluble vitamins are stored in the liver and can be toxic (especially A and D) if you go overboard on them for several months.

The water-soluble variety, taken in excess, are excreted daily in your urine. But why overwork your kidneys? Take care of them, you've got only one set!

There's no one pill (in any dosage) that will make you healthy. The factors involved in the health of any given person are so numerous that a computer would be needed to do a realistic evaluation of one's health.

Besides the possibility of a toxic effect (in the long run) with large doses of vitamins (natural or synthetic), overdosing on supplements can also cut the fat off your wallet in no time.

NATURAL OR SYNTHETIC?

Is there a difference between a natural vitamin and a synthetic one?

Some experts say yes and some say no—as long as the potency is equal, of course. For example, 300 mg of synthetic vitamin C is equal to 300 mg of natural vitamin C. But there is still the question of assimilation: Are natural vitamins better absorbed by the body than synthetic ones? And if they are, would one need a higher potency of synthetic vitamin to get the same benefits as with natural vitamins? The debate goes on.

Many people consume synthetic vitamins without knowing it. The fact that you're buying vitamins from a natural food store instead of a local drugstore is no guarantee that you're getting the natural product. For example, most vitamin B and C on the market today is synthetic.

The best advice I can give you as to whether you should go the natural or synthetic route is to try both forms of supplements, and then you be the judge.

HOW TO BUY, TAKE, AND TEST SUPPLEMENTS

So you've finally decided to take food supplements after considering the facts. Congratulations! It's a smart move. You can't go wrong from now on—or can you?

You can go wrong. Buying food supplements is not much different from buying any other product on the market. That's why you have to buy the best food supplements available. And generally speaking the best in anything costs more.

Although you don't have to look for the most expensive line of supplements on sale when looking for a reliable food supplement company, do shoot for the ones that keep their prices within the upper range bracket and that are not afraid to offer you extensive, detailed literature (pamphlets) on

Food Supplements

their line of supplements. Beware of cheaper-priced bottles of vitamins with fancy designs on the label that tell you nothing except to take one tablet a day. If only these were on the market, I wouldn't take any supplements at all.

Okay, suppose you have found a good, reliable company, and you have bought a variety of their products to sample. So when's the best time to take supplements and how should they be taken? The best time for a dieter to take his supplements is after breakfast. Why? The reason is twofold. First, if you take them only once a day as an after-breakfast morning-ritual, the chances that you'll forget them are practically nil, especially after the habit is well established. The best way not to forget them at first is to keep your supplements in sight: on a wall shelf, on the kitchen table, or any place else where you are sure not to miss them. Second, if you take such supplements as wheat germ oil and desiccated liver, the calories and particularly the energy they yield will serve you best through the day when you need them (certainly not before going to bed when you're idle).

Protein supplements are the exception to the rule. Serving mainly to build and repair the body tissues and being relatively low in calories, protein powder and amino acid tablets can be used effectively after lunch or dinner (to keep your blood-sugar normal so you won't crave for sweets all evening long).

I read in a health magazine that one way to find out if the supplements you take are well assimilated in the body is to drop many different tablets in a glass of hot water and to let them soak for half an hour. The tablets that are not dissolved after that time won't be assimilated by your system. Or so goes the theory. But don't take that for granted; the hydrochloric acid in your stomach cannot be compared to hot water—such acid can dissolve almost anything. (Michael Lotito of Grenoble, France, has eaten bicycles and TV sets without ever upsetting his stomach.) One sure way to know your supplements haven't been assimilated is when you find a complete tablet in your stool. Otherwise don't even think about it.

Nature works best when not disturbed. But don't forget to relax for 15 minutes after each meal. That's the best start toward good assimilation.

Basically, there are two ways to test a supplement: on a short-term basis (about a week) to test your compatibility with the product and on a long-term basis to test how your energy level and your health in general is being affected. Within the first week of taking a new product (you have to test supplements one at a time), if you experience a reaction such as stomach pain, headache, dizziness or swelling, stop immediately. It could be a major allergy to the basic components of the supplement or a minor allergy due to the binders in the tablet, or both. Wait a week and then resume taking the product. Do this a couple of times. If you experience negative reactions each time you're on the supplement, discard it. Then start taking another supplement and see what it does for you. When the initial testing goes without problems, keep taking the new supplement for at least two months. All along, make mental notes of how you feel in the following situations: when you wake up in the morning, when you come home after having worked overtime, when you finish exercising, and when you go to bed at night. Also look for any changes in your hair, eyes, and skin. Do you recuperate faster after physical or emotional stress? In short, look for clues that indicate a positive reaction to the product.

It could take well over a month before you will observe any positive effects from a particular supplement, and such changes, unlike the strong negative reactions from synthetic supplements, are subtle in nature. Moreover, if you start taking two or three new supplements at the same time, you'll never know which one is doing what.

No one can test a dietary supplement as well as you can. Basic physiology is the same for all human beings but everyone has his own peculiarities which must be taken into account in evaluating a supplement. If your best friend thrives on desiccated liver tablets but you get indigestion each time you take the product, forget it. Try something else instead, such as wheat germ oil capsules or blackstrap molasses.

A final word of warning: Never take your supplements on an empty stomach, particularly in the morning and especially vitamin C, which can cause heartburn. Always take supplements after breakfast. Or if you don't have breakfast, take them after lunch or dinner. A supplement is something to be added to complete a thing, an extension to strengthen the whole, and not the other way around.

We should take the magic out of health food supplements and regard them for what they really are: a long-term insurance on health that could reduce medical bills and increase energy by more than *20 percent*. Nothing else. But then that's a lot.

RATING THE SUPPLEMENTS

Following and in alphabetical order is an appraisal of the most popular dietary supplements on the market. The ratings are based on my own experience with those products at different times and in a variety of dosages, plus feedback from members who trained at my gym. Incidentally, most of them reported a marked loss of energy when they trained for a long stretch without taking any supplements. Whether or not food supplements work on the basis of mind over matter—known as the placebo effect—is debatable. Research in this field is still in the dark ages. I think the positive effects of food supplements are in large part physiological. Such supplements as wheat germ oil, vitamin E, and desiccated liver have been scientifically tested and proven highly effective. Others have been found ineffective due to their insufficient natural potencies, and some products are too new on the market to report any established long-term benefits.

In a health food store you can find just about any substitute to the food you usually buy at the grocery store, including chips and pizza. We will deal here only with supplements per se.

Amino Acid Tablets

Amino acids are the essential components of protein. There are 22 amino acids. Fourteen are called non-essential and can be manufactured by the body. The remaining eight are called essential and must come from the food we eat. Their main functions are the building and mending of the body tissue, and they also produce energy. The advantage of amino acids over protein powder is that they are predigested; they get into the blood stream faster and use less energy to do so. Although they are more expensive than protein powder, they are worth it. They should be used after meals to help you keep your blood-sugar normal, thus reducing your overall hunger. Recommended.

Bran

Bran bought on the market is the outer coating of cereals—usually wheat. It's probably the most inexpensive food supplement available today. By giving you more fiber in your diet, it can improve your digestion and your intestinal evacuation. Thus, it's especially effective against constipation. But be careful not to eat too much bran, particularly if you're a vegetarian because it can drain zinc out of your blood before it can be metabolized. One teaspoonful every other day is enough. Take one tablespoonful daily if you're constipated. It's been taken with juice, yogurt, or sprinkled on cereals. Recommended.

Bone Meal

A white, coarse powder, resulting from crushing and grinding of veal bones. A good supplier of calcium and phosphorous. Available in tablets too. Almost tasteless and easy to digest, this supplement promotes healthy teeth and bones. Recommended.

Blackstrap Molasses

A dark, thick syrup, rich in minerals (especially potassium) and in natural carbohydrates. Best taken with skim milk or juice. Since it's a concentrated product, use it sparingly. One teaspoonful a day is sufficient; preferably taken at breakfast. Recommended.

Collagen (Liquid Protein)

Collagen is obtained by boiling (hydrolisis) cartilage and connective tissues of animals. The result is a thick, dark and *terrible tasting* syrup that has to be flavored heavily to conceal its taste. Even then it tastes awful. Collagen is an incomplete protein to which manufacturers add synthetic tryptophan (an essential amino acid). To top the cake it's an expensive supplement and it can produce heartburn. Not recommended.

Note: A few years ago the Food and Drug Administration reported on deaths apparently due to the almost exclusive use of this product in an effort to lose weight. Any supplement or any food used exclusively over a long period of time can cause severe malnutrition and death.

Desiccated Liver

Desiccated liver is regular liver that is dried out, pulverized into powder, and compressed into tablets. Liver is about 60 percent protein and contains all the essential amino acids. It's a good source of vitamin A, B complex, D, as well as minerals, such as iron, copper, and calcium.

Desiccated liver has many advantages over regular liver. The water and its impurities have been removed, so has the fat. But all the nutrients are preserved. Moreover, a red protein pigment found in desiccated liver by Dr. Minor J. Coon of University of Michigan was shown to improve the ability of the body to get rid of fatigue toxins. An experiment with rats showed that the group fed on desiccated liver swam almost ten times as long as the group that received none. You should buy only Argentinian defatted liver. Recommended.

Dolomite

This supplement is a mineral that is rich in magnesium and calcium. It comes in white or gray tablets. But being *inorganic* it's not well assimilated by the body and it usually contains high levels of lead. Not recommended.

Digestive Tablets

There are many kinds of digestive tablets on the market. They are made of different enzymes that act on the metabolism of fats, protein, and carbohydrates. But the body already supplies those enzymes in digestion. You don't need to take them in tablets. Not recommended.

If you have digestion problems don't take pills. Find the cause. Stop smoking, eat better, do some exercise, and lay down for 15 minutes after each meal. In this way, you will rehabilitate your digestive system.

Ginseng

This forked root plant (Panax Ginseng) from eastern Asia is believed to have medicinal properties. Ginseng is not a concentrated supplement and the vitamins and minerals it contains are not potent enough to produce any appreciable effect. As for the supposed aphrodisiac qualities ginseng can yield, forget it. The only *real* aphrodisiac known to man is *desire*. So considering the price tag it carries, ginseng is quite overrated. Not recommended.

Garlic

Garlic may well be the best thing we have to fight the common cold. It is also believed to be effective in reducing blood pressure. Containing vitamin C, calcium, magnesium, potassium, and sulfur, garlic is also rich in mineral salts. Laboratory researchers have also shown that garlic has true antibacterial properties.

In the heydays of his body-building glory, my brother (who swore by garlic) used to remind me that if eating garlic helped the Egyptians build those wonderful pyramids, it was good enough for him. Impressed by so much faith, I started taking garlic too. Unfortunately this product has a big olfactive drawback that can mean bad breath, unless you know how to take it. Here is the secret: Take garlic only before going to bed, and for each garlic oil capsule you take make sure you also get one chlorophyll tablet—the magnesium in chlorophyll acts as a deodorant. Recommended.

Glandular Products

A few years ago, products made from desiccated glands such as adrenal, pituitary, pancreas, and kidney invaded the market. In their publicity, manufacturers subtly claimed that the products are natural substitutes for steroids. However, glandular products cannot endanger your health, but I don't think they're worth their costly price. Not recommended.

Kelp

From those big, brown seaweeds come tablets known as kelp. This supplement is mostly taken for its minerals (over 40 of them). Never take kelp in large doses (ten to thirty tablets) in the belief that it can activate your thyroid gland and thus help you reduce your body weight. It could produce the opposite effect. Kelp taken internally is an excellent hair conditioner. It can also prevent or even *reduce* grayish hair. Recommended.

Lecithin

Occurring in all plant and animal tissues, lecithin is usually produced commercially from soybeans. Lecithin is found in the brain, liver, kidney, and heart; it's a combination of fatty acids. Lecithin keeps your nerves and skin in good health.

You can buy lecithin in granules or in capsules. Not recommended. Lecithin is better assimilated when you get it through regular foods.

Protein Powder

The number of protein powders available today is staggering. You have to be selective in your choice. Quality in protein is determined by the P.E.R. (Protein Efficiency Ratio). The highest quality protein comes from egg white with P.E.R. of 3.9.* Soya protein rates 1.7. Between these ratings is meat protein with a P.E.R. of 3.3 and milk protein yielding 2.8.

The best protein powder is made from 100 percent eggs, or milk and eggs. Soya protein is not as good; it is incomplete and hard to digest because it's usually uncooked. Most good protein powders are free of carbohydrates and fat. Beware of protein powders that are filled with yeast (why pay the price of protein if it's yeast you want), or of milk and egg protein that doesn't mention the amount of eggs it contains—you should strive for 25 percent. Don't waste your money on regular protein tablets. Why pay for the binder? And who wants to swallow so many tablets in a day? You can mix protein powder with half a glass of water at the end of a meal or with fruit juice; however, don't use protein powder too liberally because even protein, if taken in excess (unused calories), can be converted to fat by the body. Recommended. A good asset in losing weight.

Pollen

Bee pollen is harvested by the bee on flowers. It's the male element in fertilization. Pollen contains amino acids, vitamins, sugar, and mineral salt but in negligible amounts. Some athletes, runners in particular, are great believers in its stamina-building quality. As far as I'm concerned, each time I took bee pollen (one tablespoonful of granules), I experienced a weird, upsetting feeling in my stomach. Besides, it's too costly. For half the

---

*The egg white P.E.R. (3.9) is equal to a net utilization value of about .90.

price of a small bottle of bee pollen, I can have the same funny feeling in my stomach on the roller coaster. Not recommended.

Royal Jelly

Another overrated supplement. Highly prized by some people (especially the manufacturers of the product), royal jelly is a substance secreted in the pharyngeal glands of worker bees. It's impressive to learn that queen bees live an average of five years compared to forty-five days for worker bees (royal jelly is the sole food of queen bees). But a laboratory examination of royal jelly reveals an *infinitesimal* amount of nutrients which aren't worth writing home about. Besides, it's an expensive supplement. Having tested royal jelly extensively before competitions—without any positive result—I don't recommend this product.

RNA and DNA

Ribonucleic acid and deoxyribonucleic acid are two complex compounds found in all living cells. In relation to your body's needs and how easily you can get it from regular food, buying this costly supplement (capsules) is ridiculous. Definitely not recommended.

Vitamin A

Vitamin A is needed for healthy skin and keen eyesight. It helps the body fight infection and speeds the healing of wounds. Vitamin A is found mostly in liver, egg yolk, and fish liver oils. Green and yellow vegetables provide carotene, which is later converted to vitamin A. For natural supplements, the best sources are halibut liver oil and beta carotene tablets.

Vitamin B Complex

Vitamin B complex is divided as follows:
B1 (thiamine),
B2 (riboflavin), niacin, pantothenic acid,
B6 (pyridoxine), biotin, folic acid and
B12 (cyanocobalamin).

It's not a good idea to take these vitamins separately in the form of supplements because all B vitamins work together. If you take too much of an isolated B vitamin you can create a shortage of another B vitamin. Can we assume, therefore, that taking a tablet of B complex (containing all of the B's) is better? No, because all B vitamins on the market (including health food stores) are synthetic. Definitely not recommended.

Note: Vitamin B complex promotes a healthy nervous system and skin, as well as good vision; it also helps metabolize proteins, fat, carbohydrates, and helps maintain a normal hemoglobin. The best sources (besides regular foods) of natural vitamin B complex are raw wheat germ and desiccated liver.

Vitamin C

The hold of this important vitamin on the public mind is incredible. The discovery of vitamin C's scurvy-curing properties and the much-publicized work of Nobel Prize winner Linus Pauling on vitamin C and the common cold are responsible in great part for this phenomenon. Vitamin C, also known as ascorbic acid, promotes healthy gums, helps your organism resist infection, and strengthens the capillaries. Most vitamin C tablets on the market today are synthetic. Not recommended. The good news is that all vitamins act as catalysts in the body. Thus vitamin C is needed in small amounts and can be obtained from such foods as tomatoes, cantaloupe, kiwi fruit, broccoli, and potatoes.

Vitamin D

Vitamin D helps build strong bones and teeth and promotes calcium assimilation. Your body can produce it when bare skin is exposed to sun rays. As a supplement, it is recommended in the form of fish-liver oil.

Vitamin E

Vitamin E (tocopherol) acts as an antioxidant and helps keep the reproducing organs in good health. Natural sources are wheat germ, nuts, and vegetables. As a supplement, look for D-alpha Tocopherol (DL-Alpha Tocopherol means it's synthetic). Recommended.

Wheat Germ

Wheat germ doesn't require much introduction. It's a good source of vitamin B complex, E, and F, and it has some proteinic values. Keep wheat germ in the refrigerator, or it will become rancid. Use it in yogurt, oatmeal, or sprinkle the flakes on anything you want. You can even eat it as a cereal with skim milk and sliced bananas. Delicious, easy to digest, and inexpensive. Highly recommended. Buy fresh raw wheat germ, not the roasted variety.

Wheat Germ Oil

Wheat germ oil is regarded as a classic among food supplements, particularly by athletes. The work of Dr. Thomas K. Cureton on wheat germ oil is well established. He showed that a person can increase his stamina by 51 percent with only one teaspoonful of wheat germ oil taken daily while following a regular exercise program.

Keep your bottle of wheat germ oil tightly closed in the fridge. Take one teaspoonful daily after breakfast. Highly recommended.

Yeast

Brewer's yeast is used in brewing. It's a mass of microscopic plants. Brewer's yeast is about 50 percent protein and contains B complex vitamins. This supplement has many drawbacks. The taste is so bitter that nothing can hide it; it causes fermentation of carbohydrates often resulting in gas and indigestion; it is too high in phosphorous (you have plenty of this electronegative mineral from the meat products); and it can even cause allergies. Not recommended.

Note: Torula yeast is even worse. You can end up with liver problems because of the way it's cultivated.

Zinc

Zinc is a mineral that has received plenty of publicity lately. It is said to cure about every illness known to human beings, particularly prostate problems. There's no denying that zinc is needed by the body but it's needed only in extremely small doses; it's a trace mineral. If you eat a wide variety of foods, you don't have to worry about getting enough zinc. Liver, shellfish, and meats are especially rich sources of zinc.

Not recommended as a supplement.

31

SPECIAL INSTRUCTIONS

There is no use whatever trying to help people who do not help themselves. You cannot push anyone up a ladder unless he be willing to climb himself.
(Andrew Carnegie)

Don't jump into the Cheater's Diet as if there were no tomorrow. The wisest thing you could do is to wait two or three days before embarking on the Cheater's Diet. Why? As a gym owner, I often saw men and women start their diet and exercise program in a frantic, bragging, watch-me-now approach, and they usually ended up throwing in the towel a few weeks later. Perhaps these people created too much pressure on themselves, and the idea of having to live up to those expectations probably defeated their well-intentioned purpose right from the onset.

On the other hand, I have observed many low-keyed persons who started on the same program and who transformed their appearance within a few short months. These people, as a group, even if they didn't show as much excitement in their initial approach, were nevertheless more determined in the long run. Also their idea of transforming their body wasn't a spur-of-the-moment impulse; it had grown in the back of their mind over a long period of time. Just as a wise runner won't start a long race full blast, you can't rush into the Cheater's Diet and expect to come out a winner.

So, if you don't start right away, what should you do? You will use those few days to let your enthusiasm build up *slowly* inside of you; but you should always keep it under control. You must think about how you will use the Cheater's Diet—all that time and at all times thereafter. But don't talk about it; your determination will be stronger. In this way, you will develop the one quality that all achievers have in common: *patience*.

You should also use that time to establish in your mind the importance of what you will do to your body. Shedding the extra weight you painfully carry around is a matter of commitment: a lifelong commitment. That's a big statement. But then you do have to keep the weight off forever and stay healthy in the process. The philosophy behind the Cheater's Diet is holistic in nature, not merely losing X amount of pounds in X amount of days.

Now, to be more concrete, let's say you've finished reading the Cheater's Diet on Sunday night, You must determine in advance how many days you will take to concentrate on your new approach to dieting. OK, say you decide to take three days to focus your mental energy into an experience that will most likely change your life. So you will start Thursday morning.

In those three days, the technique you will use is simply a form of self-hypnosis or psyching as weighlifters call it. Psyche means *breath, life,* and *soul*. That's what you have to instill in yourself before you start on this new diet. Have you ever watched a weightlifter as he prepares himself to lift a weight? Unlike in tennis where you have two chances to serve and endless sets, a weightlifter has only three attempts at making a lift. And each attempt better be successful for the tremendous energy involved in each lift is incredible. It's a do-or-die situation each time the weightlifter approaches the bar. There are no two ways about it; the bar can only go *up*. Otherwise months and even years of effort will be reduced to nothing. You have to psych yourself in those three pre-diet days with the same intensity that a weightlifter would put into concentration before a lift. As often as you can, "see" yourself getting confidently and smoothly into the Cheater's Diet on that particular day you have planned. Visualize the control you *will have* over the whole situation. Imagine what you *will look like* once you reach your desired weight, what you *will do* with your new body and with that extra vitality. To conclude: For those three days eat what you want, drink what you want, but try to stay in a familiar environment; relax your body and focus your mental power on your goal of losing weight until it becomes an obsession.

If you have done your homework as you should, you will be so filled with the importance of your project that you won't sleep much the night before you start.

That's the frame of mind you should put your spirit in.

Now you're ready to go. It's the day. The one you have dreamed about. In fact, you just took your first meal according to the Cheater's Diet's precepts and already you think about the forbidden goodies you will eat four days later. You can hardly wait: you will cheat regularly, you will enjoy cheating without feeling guilty and you will lose weight. And moreover, considering that you will have only one cheating meal out of every twelve to sixteen regular meals, you will be as healthy as anyone can be.

But don't be too impatient. Your body will need a few weeks, or even more, to adjust to your new way of eating, depending on how out of shape you are to begin with. Forget about writing down what you eat, weighing foods, etc. Rely on your body instinct—you literally *feel it* when you have lost weight. Be confident in the outcome. I'm sure you will thrive on the Cheater's Diet because it is the *only* permanent way I know to keep your weight down and your health up without parting with all the joy of gourmet cuisine.

I remember once I was waiting in line at a well-known fried chicken eatery (mind you, it was a scheduled cheating meal). Right in front of me stood this tough-looking man. He had about 200 lbs. of fat on him. He was wearing a black tank top and was munching a big cigar. Across the right shoulder, a worn-out tattoo read: *I've loved, I've been hurt, now I know.* This impressed me. I would never have the guts to walk around with such a statement tattooed on my body, but that's not the point. I think that the poor guy must have been an unsuccessful ex-dieter and might as well have on his left shoulder another tattoo that reads: I've lost weight, I've gained it back, now I don't know.

As far as I'm concerned, any kind of tattoo is out. But if you prize them as much as the Cheater's Diet and you intend to get one anywhere on your body, may I suggest this one: *I've cheated, I've lost, now I love myself.*

Many people have a book lurking inside them, ready to jump on paper, set free by a will and a pen. At last, after nearly ten years, mine is out. I think my book, *The Cheater's Diet*, fills a need in the dietary battlefield for it unveils a new approach to control people's weight in a healthy and permanent way.

The war against fat is far from over, but with the Cheater's Diet and the right dose of indulgence, plus a positive attitude, I know you will succeed—once and for all.

More power to the *new* you.

IF NOT NOW, WHEN?

IF NOT I, WHO?

(Chinese Proverb)

INDEX

A

Age, health and, 120
Alcoholic beverages, 100
American diet:
    average meal, 37–38
    fast-food eaters, 39
    health-food fanatics, 39
    vegetarians, 38
Amino acid tablets, 147
Amphetamines, 62–63
Anabolism, 6
Anemia:
    desiccated liver for, 133
    vegetarianism and, 38
Appetite, definition of, 20
Argentinian liver, 132–133, 148
Arthritis, 132
Asparagus sauce, 88
Asparagus du Tremblay, 85
Aspic-o-veggies, 85

B

Banana, dietary myth about, 28
Bathing, 122
Binges, compulsive eater, 46
Blackstrap molasses, 31, 148
    in juices, 100
Body building, Cheater's Diet and, 33–34
Body types, 36–37
Body wrap, 24
Bone meal, 147
Bran, 147
Bread:
    in Cheater's Diet, 70–71
    dietary myth about, 27–28
Breakfast:
    recipes for, 88–90
    sample menu, 76
Breakfast of champions, 89

Breathing, 125–127
Brussels sprouts royal, 85–86
Butter, dietary myth about, 30

C

Cabbage fruit salad, 86
Caffein, 101
Calories, 11–17
    calorie chart of common foods, 14–17
    in Cheater's Diet, 68–69
    excess of, 13–14
    fat, 12
    food sources and, 12–13
Carbohydrates, 11
Casserole amandine, 82
Catabolism, 6
Cellulite:
    smoking and, 104–105
    water and, 102
Cereals, in Cheater's Diet, 70–71
Cheap-grocery breakfast, 88–89
Cheap-grocery-breakfast drink, 88
Cheater's brochette, 82
Cheater's casserole, 81
Cheater's diet (*see also* Cheating meals)
    body building and, 33–34
    bread-cereal group in, 70–71
    calories in, 68–69
    cheating, 93–98
    drinks, 99–102
    eating out and, 110–113
    exercise, 124–130
    food allergies and, 107
    food chart (allowed and forbidden foods), 72–75
    food substitution, 72
    getting started, 154–156
    hospitalization and, 107–108
    meals per day, 75–76
    meals per day, sample menu, 76–77
    meal substitutes, 108–109

Cheater's diet *(cont'd)*
  meat group in, 69–70
  milk-cheese group in, 71
  modifications for, 106–109
  monitoring weight, 114–118
  origin of, 66–67
  recipes, 80–92
  sample menu, 92
  seasonings, guide, 77–80
  showering and, 122
  sweeteners in, 31
  testing of, 67–68
  time span of, 31
  uniqueness of, 33
  vegetable-fruit group in, 70
Cheater's mini breakfast, 90
Cheater's potatoes, 85
Cheater's quiche, 83
Cheater's sauce, 87
Cheating con carne, 82–83
Cheating meals, 93–98
  best time for, 96
  effective cheating, 97
  frustration preventing techniques, 95
  junk food guide, 98
  rationale for, 94, 97
Cheese, in Cheater's Diet, 71
Cholesterol, dietary myth about, 29–30
Choline/inositol combination, 25
Cinnamon oatmeal, 90
Coffee, 100, 132
Collagen, 148
Compulsive eater, 46–48
Control, over life pressure, 122–123
Cottage a la mode, 89
Creams and lotions, weight loss products, 25

D

Desiccated liver tablets, 142
  for anemia, 133
  explanation of, 148
  fatigue and, 132,
Desserts, recipes for, 91
Dieters, tips for dieters, 134–139 *(see also* Eating profiles)
Diets:
  eating less, 18
  failure of, 34
  individuality and, 19
  juices and, 34
  most popular, 9
  rules of good diet, 9–10

Digestive tablets, 148
Dinner, sample menu, 77
Diuretics, 63
  vitamin C, 25
DNA, 151
Dolomite, 148
Dressing du chef, 87
Dressings, recipes for, 86–88
Drinks, 99–102
  alcoholic beverages, 100
  coffee/tea, 100
  juice, 101–102
  liquids allowed, 99
  meal substitutes, 108–109
  recipes for, 91–92
  soft drinks, 100
  soup, 101
  water, 101
du Tremblay pot-au-feu, 80–81
du Tremblay special dressing, 87

E

Eating, single foods, 31–32, 34
Eating binges, 36
Eating habits, parental influences, 4
Eating preferences, 38
Eating profiles, 36–39
  compulsive eater, 46–48
  food insecurity, 44–45
  ignorant dieter, 52–54
  lazy dieter, 49–51
  of lonely person, 41–42
  on-and-off dieter, 55–56
Ectomorph, 36–37
Eggs, dietary myth about, 29–30
Emotional stress, exercise and, 129
Emulsifiers, natural fat emulsifiers, 24–25
Endomorph, 36–37
Energy:
  formula for, 132
  movement and, 125
Environment, influence on weight, 3
Exercise, 124–130
  best types, 127–128
  breathing, 125–127
  Cheater's Diet and, 33–34
  duration of session, 128
  emotional stress and, 129
  heartbeat and, 128–129
  pseudo-exercise, 127
  self-image and, 130
  skin resilience and, 129
Exotic fruit salad, 86

Index

F

Fast-food eater, 39
Fasting, 58–61
  disadvantages of, 58–59
  one-day fast, 59–61
Fat-cell theory, 30
Fat emulsifiers, 24–25
Fats, calories in, 11, 12
Fatigue, desiccated liver tablets and, 132
Fat-soluble vitamins, 143–144
Fiber, digestion of, 12
Fiesta salad, 86
Fillet de sole amandine, 84
Fish, 70
Food, components of, 11
Food allergies, Cheater's Diet modification for, 107
Food chart, allowed and forbidden foods, 72–75
Food combinations, 33
Food groups, in Cheater's Diet, 69–71
Food labels, reading of, 20–22
Food substitution, in Cheater's Diet, 72
Food supplements, 140–153
  amino acid tablets, 147
  best time for, 146
  bran, 147
  bone meal, 147
  blackstrap molasses, 148
  buying of, 144–145
  collagen, 148
  desiccated liver, 148
  digestive tablets, 148–149
  dolomite, 148
  DNA, 151
  explanation of, 141
  garlic, 149
  ginseng, 149
  glandular products, 149
  kelp, 149–150
  lecithin, 150
  megadose, 143–144
  necessity of, 140–141
  protein powder, 150
  pollen, 150–151
  rating, most common supplements, 146–153
  royal jelly, 151
  RNA, 151
  testing of, 145–146
  vitamin A, 151
  vitamin B complex, 151–152
  vitamin C, 152
  vitamin D, 152
  vitamin E, 152

Food supplements (cont'd)
  vitamins, 143–144
  wheat germ, 152
  wheat germ oil, 152–153
  yeast, 153
  zinc, 153
Formic acid, in honey, 31
Francis' dressing, 87–88
French toast a la Tremblay, 89
Friends, monitoring weight and, 117–118
Fruits, in Cheater's Diet, 70
Frustration, prevention techniques, 95

G

Garlic, 149
Ginseng, 149
Glandular products, 149
Good supplements, 65
Gout, 9
Grape punch, 92
Grapefruit, dietary myth about, 28–29

H

Health:
  age and, 120
  salt and, 121
  sugar and, 121–122
Health-food fanatic, 38
Heartbeat, exercise and, 128–129
Herbal tea, 100–101
Herbs, 78–79
Honey, unpasteurized, 31
Hospital, stay in, 107–108
Hot potato sauce, 87
Hunger, definition of, 20
Hypertension, 129

I

Injections, for fat loss, 63–64
Insecurity, food, 44–45

J

Juices, 101–102
  diets and, 34
Junk food:
  cheating meals, 68
  in health food stores, 39
Junk food guide, 98

K

Kelp, 149–150

L

Lacto-vegetarian, 38
Lazy dieters, 49–51
Lecithin, 150
  in egg yolk, 29–30
Liquid protein, 148
Loneliness, obesity and, 41–42
Lunch, sample menu, 76–77

M

Macrobiotic dieting, 38
Main dishes, recipes for, 80–84
Margarine, dietary myth about, 30
Massage, 24
Meals:
  meal substitutes, 108–109
  of single foods, 31–32, 34
Meat, in Cheater's Diet, 69–70
Megadose, 143–144
Men, body fat of, 4
Menstruation, body weight and, 19–20
Mesomorph, 36–37
Metabolism, 6–7
  body types and, 37
  slowing with age, 7
Milk, in Cheater's Diet, 71
Milkshakes, meal substitutes, 108–109
Minted carrots, 84
Mirrors, monitoring weight, 116–117
Modified Cheater's Diet, 106–109
Movement, energy and, 124

N

Natural flavorings, 79
Nuts, 70

O

Obesity:
  eating binges, 36
  environmental influences, 3
  health and, 41
  limitations of, 40–41
  loneliness and, 41–42

Obesity (cont'd)
  parental habits and, 4
  sex differences and, 4–5 (see also Eating profiles)
Oil, 132
Omelette Claudine, 81–82
Omelette souffle a la vanille, 91
Orange juice, 132
Oven-warm breakfast, 90
Ovo-vegetarian, 38

P

Pancakes, 70–71
Parents, influence on weight, 4
Parties, dieting and, 111–112
Pasta, 25
  in Cheater's Diet, 70
Photographs, monitoring weight, 117
Pineapple, dietary myth about, 29
Pollen, 150–151
Potatoes, dietary myth about, 28
Pressure:
  inward, 122
  outward, 122–123
Protein, 11
  liquid, 148
  overconsumption of, 9
Protein powder, 150

R

Recipes, 80–92
  asparagus sauce, 88
  asparagus du Tremblay, 85
  aspic-o-veggies, 85
  breakfast of champions, 89
  brussels sprouts royal, 85–86
  cabbage fruit salad, 86
  casserole amandine, 82
  cheap-grocery breakfast, 88–89
  cheap-grocery-breakfast drink, 88
  cheater's brochette, 82
  cheater's casserole, 81
  cheater's mini breakfast, 90
  cheater's potatoes, 85
  cheater's quiche, 83
  cheater's sauce, 87
  cheating con carne, 82–83
  cinnamon oatmeal, 90
  cottage a la mode, 89
  dressing du chef, 87

Index

Recipes (cont'd)
  du Tremblay pot-au-feu, 80–81
  du Tremblay special dressing, 87
  exotic fruit salad, 86
  fiesta salad, 86
  fillet de sole amandine, 84
  Francis' dressing, 87–88
  French toast a la Tremblay, 89
  grape punch, 92
  hot potato sauce, 87
  meal substitutes, 108–109
  minted carrots, 84
  omelette Claudine, 81–82
  omelette souffle a la vanille, 91
  oven-warm breakfast, 90
  Red Baron dressing, 88
  rice 'n' nice, 83
  shrimp sauce, 88
  strawberry surprise, 91
  stuffed tomatoes, 84–85
  summer party punch, 91
  sure-cure hangover breakfast, 90
  three-star dressing, 86
  tropical punch, 91
  veal-o-veggies, 84
Restaurants, dieting and eating out, 110–111
RNA, 151
Royal jelly, 151

S

Salt, white killer, 121
Sauces, recipes for, 86–88
Sauna, 23–24
Scale, monitoring weight, 114–115
Seasonings guide, for Cheater's Diet, 77–80
Self-image, exercise and, 130
Sex differences, weight and, 4–5
Sex, obesity and, 40
Showering, 122
Shrimp sauce, 88
Side dishes, recipes for, 84–86
Smoking, 103–105
  cellulite and, 104–105
  vitamin C and, 104
  ways to stop, 105
Soft drinks, 100
Soup, 101
Spices, 78
Starch blockers, 25–26
Starches, benefits of, 25

Strawberry surprise, 91
Stretch marks, remedy for, 132
Stuffed tomatoes, 84–85
Sugar, white killer, 122
Summer party punch, 91
Sure-cure hangover breakfast, 90
Surgery, removing fat, 64
Sweeteners, honey, 31
Sweets, craving for, 32

T

Tape measures, monitoring weight, 115–116
Tea, 100, 132
  herbal tea, 100–101
Teenagers, obese, 32
Three-star dressing, 86
Tropical punch, 91

U

Uric acid, 9

V

Vacations, dieting and, 112–113
Veal-o-veggies, 84
Vegetables, in Cheater's Diet, 70
Vegetarian, 38
Vitamin A, 151
Vitamin B complex, 151–152
Vitamin C, 152
  as diuretic, 25
  smoking and, 104
Vitamin D, 152
Vitamin E, 152
Vitamins:
  fat-soluble, 143–144
  function of, 143
  mixing of, 33
  natural vs. synthetic, 144
  water-soluble, 144

W

Walking, 127
Water, 101
  cellulite and, 102
Water-soluble vitamins, 144

Weight loss:
  speed of, 32
  vs. fat loss, 19–20
Wheat germ, 152
Wheat germ capsule, 142
Wheat germ oil, 152
White killers, salt/sugar, 121–122
Whole wheat bread, reading the label, 21
Women, body fat of, 4

Y

Yeast, 153

Z

Zinc, 153